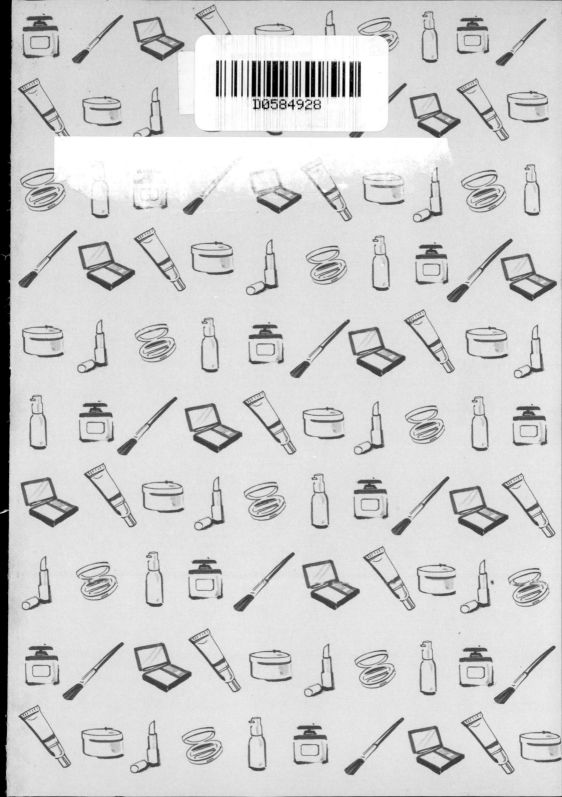

'There is a growing acceptance of aesthetic surgery in the UK, particularly in the areas of facial rejuvenation and body contouring. Consumers need accurate information to provide them with an idea of what surgical procedures can achieve, and to help them sort through the myriad options and alternatives. Plastic Makes Perfect offers helpful resources for the public and promotes sensible and safe decision-making.'

Barry M. Jones, FRCS, Past President British Association of Aesthetic Plastic Surgeons (BAAPS), Hunterian Professor RCS Eng., author of *Facial Aesthetic Surgery: A Practical Guide.*

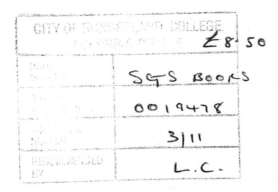

Plastic Makes Perfect

The Complete Cosmetic Beauty Guide

Wendy Lewis

First published in Great Britain in 2007 by
Orion Books
an imprint of the Orion Publishing Group Ltd
Orion House, 5 Upper St Martin's Lane,
London WC2H 9EA
An Hachette Livre UK Company

1 3 5 7 9 10 8 6 4 2

A CIP catalogue record for this book is
available from the British Library.

ISBN-13: 9780 75288 839 2

Jacket and inside illustrations by
Jacqueline Bisset

Printed in Italy by Printer Trento

The Orion Publishing Group's policy is to use papers that
are natural, renewable and recyclable and made from wood grown
in sustainable forests. The logging and manufacturing processes are
expected to conform to the environmental regulations of
the country of origin.

Every effort has been made to fulfil requirements with regard to
reproducing copyright material. The author and publisher will be
glad to rectify any omissions at the earliest opportunity.

www.orionbooks.co.uk

To my gorgeous daughter Eden, the most important person in my life, who continues to amaze, surprise and challenge me, and make me proud of her every day. My wonderful staff deserve a round of applause, particularly Ilana Greenberg, who is my right and left hand. I also want to thank Linda Land for her ingenuity and perseverance, which made this book a reality. To Sue Peart and John Koski, the most professional and supportive editors anyone could ever have: you and your whole team have made me feel like part of your family. I also want to thank Gillian de Bono for giving me a platform to delve into hot topics of interest. And I thank my lucky stars to have worked with the Orion women: Lisa Milton, Amanda Harris and Clare Wallis, who gave birth to this book (almost literally in one case) and had contagious enthusiasm for the project from start to finish. I send my gratitude to the always perfect Linda Chester, without whose generosity and gracious mentoring I may never have seen my first book in Harrods. Special thanks to Paula Fitzherbert of the Berkeley and her staff in the Caramel Room for taking great care of me. Finally, to the incredibly talented women I am privileged to count as my closest confidantes, Anne, Barbara, Elaine, Fran, Janice, Judi and Margot: your friendship has kept me strong. And to my mother Evelyn for everything.

Contents

Introduction:

Confessions of The Knife Coach®

When I had my facelift, I wrote in a feature called 'When a New Hairdo Just Won't Cut It Anymore' (*Financial Times How to Spend It*, 15 September 2004) that 50 was the new 40. Today I think we have surpassed that by a mile. Now 60 is the new 40. If you accept that as the new maths of ageing, then 50 must be the new 35, and 40 is the new 30, and so on. In other words, age doesn't really matter any more.

Boomers are turning 60 and they will glide into their twilight years like no other generation before them. (The remarkably lineless Dolly Parton and Cher celebrated their 60th birthdays in 2006!) There has never been a generation with access to the same nutrition, health care, education and living standards. And they are resisting the idea of looking old and fighting it every way they can. Boomers are redefining ageing as we know it and I am now one of them.

In my first book, *The Lowdown on Facelifts and Other Wrinkle Remedies* (Quadrille, 2000), I started Chapter 1 with creams, sailed through peels and lasers, and dived into fillers and Botox®, but I did not get into real surgery until well into Chapter 5, about halfway through the book. My rationale was that a lot of readers would have a go at the first few chapters, but when it came to reading about scalpels, scarring, anaesthetics, pulling and lifting, they would go pale and toss the book in a drawer somewhere, or bin it.

Seven years have passed, and the realm of available cosmetic enhancements is light years ahead. And we are truly the Botox® generation. Women all over the world have an insatiable appetite for information. They are more open to learning about everything – even the gory details of procedures they may never pluck up the nerve to have.

When I started my beauty consultancy in 1997, most of my clients were female, Caucasian, over 40, fairly affluent, living in the New York area and concerned primarily about their ageing faces. I have no typical client any more. I see a cross section of people, women and men, from age 18 to 80, from all over the world. They are barristers, professors, artists, actors, soccer mums, estate agents, tellers and Presidents of banks. And they are interested in everything from hair transplants and breast implants to lasers, lipo and lifts.

Being a New Yorker gives me a unique perspective on high-maintenance women – we wrote the book on it. The phrase 'New York minute' was originally coined by a cosmetic surgeon to describe how long his patients allow for bruising to go away. Manhattanites are programmed from an early age to hire a 'specialist'; cosmetic surgery is a topic of interest at soirées. New Yorkers are as fickle about surgeons as they are about restaurants and designers. The woman who has a two o'clock appointment for a peel will show up at noon and complain at twelve fifteen that she hasn't been seen yet. New Yorkers think nothing of bullying a receptionist to be 'squeezed in' for emergency Restylane®. If the forecast is rain, they may cancel their appointment because taxis will be in short supply.

In contrast, London women are more likely to be loyal, follow instructions religiously, keep their scheduled appointments, queue up gladly, go back to a doctor they weren't really happy with, rarely complain, and say 'thank you' even when they have been kept waiting for three hours for Botox®. Londoners are far more accepting of life's little inconveniences. Aside from the obvious cultural differences, the other variable is that there are only about 400 dermatologists and 300 plastic surgeons in the UK, so the choices are very limited. (America has around 10,000 and 6,000 respectively.)

In this beauty scripture, I have intertwined surgical procedures with what I call 'cosmetic surgery lite' – less invasive alternatives – to give you a rundown of the most popular procedures. I offer up all the facts, the good, the bad and the really bad, so that you can be empowered to make informed choices.

I have divided the options into three basic categories of treatment:

1 **Invasive** Proper surgery done to reshape or refine parts of the face and body, involving going to the hospital and an anaesthetic.
2 **Minimally invasive** Falling somewhere in between surgery with visible scars and the non-invasive category; can be performed in a doctor's surgery under a local anaesthetic.
3 **Non-invasive** Wash-and-wear injections and resurfacing treatments such as lasers and peels, as well as clinical skincare.

Most women dabble in level 3 – the foreplay phase. Some graduate to level 2, but many linger somewhere between levels 3 and 2. The process of jumping from level 3 all the way up to level 1 can often be a long one. It takes a lot more consideration and a bit more nerve to go all the way.

Cosmetic enhancements can be seductive. You should give each procedure you undertake very careful consideration so that you don't end up a cosmetic surgery victim. In this comprehensive guide, you will quickly learn that surgery is nothing like what you have seen on 'reality' television or *Nip/Tuck*. I hope it will help you to distinguish between truth and tabloid, so that you know what you are getting into before you take the plunge.

In this book I refer to cosmetic surgery patients as 'she' and doctors as 'he'. This is simply for ease of reading. Of course men too undergo cosmetic surgery and there are many good doctors working in this field who are women (but still not enough).

When it comes to having cosmetic surgery, ultimately the responsibility for whether or not to go ahead lies with you. No doctor is obliged to refuse you, even if you are not an ideal candidate. Anyone who desires cosmetic surgery will be able to get it, as long as she can pay for it. If the first consultant says no, someone else will be happy to do it. But the point is not whether or not you can have it done, it is whether or not you should, and if you should, when to have it, what to have, and who to let do it.

Before diving into *Plastic Makes Perfect*, get yourself a Post-it® Flag Highlighter. This clever invention allows you to mark pages to refer back to, and highlight anything of particular importance. There is a lot of information on these pages and I don't want you to miss out on any of it!

Cheers and happy hunting!

Wendy

GETTING UP CLOSE AND PERSONAL

Best feature: my lips
Worst feature: my hips

Desert Island beauty product A light-textured moisturiser with antioxidants or peptides and SPF 15–50. I have many favourites: there isn't just one I use every day, and I switch frequently. And I couldn't live without a creamy lipstick. At last count, I have as many lipsticks as I have shoes. I am totally brand-agnostic.

Desert Island beauty treatment I wish I had time to do all the things I'd like to do! I go for my hair colour every six weeks like clockwork, and I have my Botox® religiously every four months to smooth my forehead and crow's feet.

Favourite cosmetic surgery I have never been unhappy with what I've had done, but some things were definitely more effective than others. Having the bump taken off the bridge of my nose at the age of 23 was my first cosmetic surgery. The bump was something I had always hated, and having it removed changed my whole face. After that, having my upper eyelids done when I turned 45 was a really nice improvement.

Biggest beauty regret Not being diligent with a good fitness regime. I live a real city life, and sit in front of a laptop 14+ hours a day. Running to catch a taxi or jogging through airports is not enough to keep your thighs taut and your bottom high. I am a yo-yo dieter and that causes earlier sagging and dragging.

Cosmetic surgery wish list I would love to have my body lifted one day, but I don't think I will ever pluck up the motivation to deal with the hard recovery and long scars that would follow.

Beauty goal Looking good for my age, not older. I don't mind telling what I have had, but I never want to look 'done'.

Beauty passion Antique beauty adverts and ephemera, crystal perfume bottles, powder jars and decorative mirrors, ranging from Victorian to 1940s glamour.

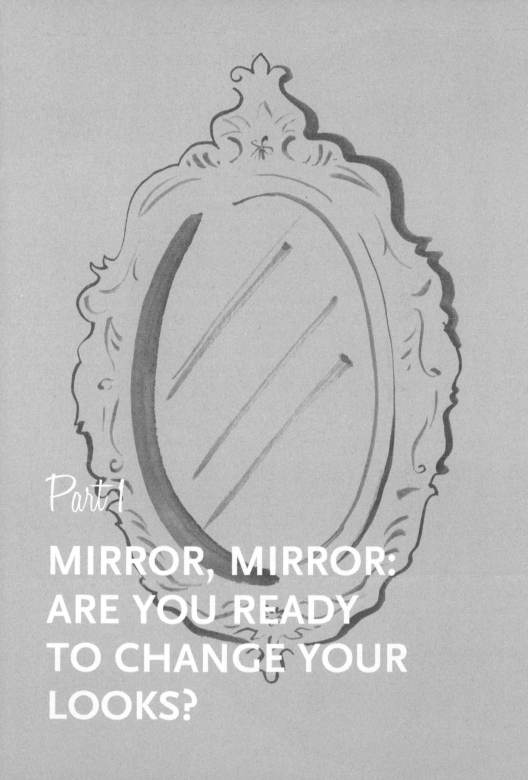

Part 1

MIRROR, MIRROR: ARE YOU READY TO CHANGE YOUR LOOKS?

1

Ageing Gracefully or Ageing Gorgeously

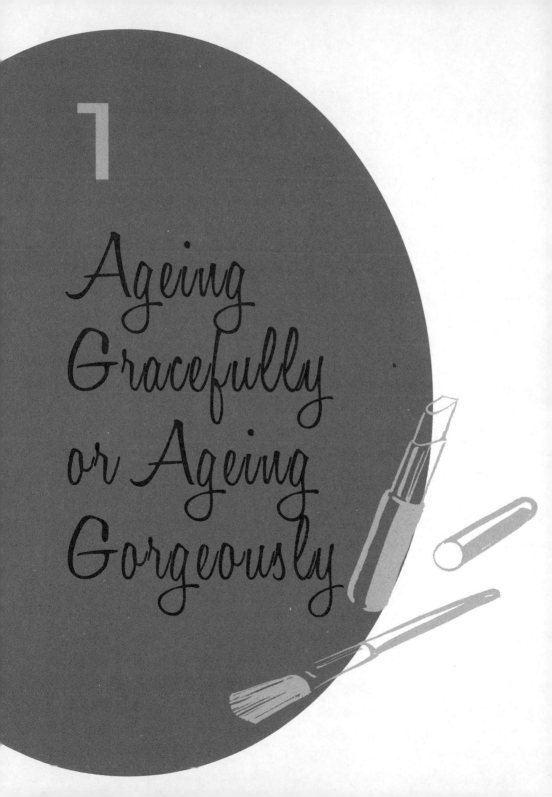

IT BEGAN WITH A NOSE

It is amazing to think that cosmetic surgery has been around for over four centuries. In 1597, Gaspare Tagliacozzi, a professor of surgery at the University of Bologna, published *De Curtorum Chirurgia per Insitionem*, an illustrated guide that documented the first nose job in history. In a woodcut, Tagliacozzi depicted a Renaissance man sans nose, with his arm extended and a flap hanging from his biceps. In another woodcut, he wears an intricate device that is strapping his arm up and back so that his face appears to be buried in his armpit and his hand is extended over his head as if he is searching for his brain. The contraption stayed on long enough for tissue from his arm to form a new nose. Tagliacozzi was the first surgeon credited with the realisation that improving a person's looks might also improve his life. He was several hundred years ahead of his time.

Sir Harold Gillies is considered the father of British plastic surgery, although he was actually a New Zealander. However, his cousin Archibald McIndoe is the most renowned. Also born in New Zealand, McIndoe moved to England in 1931 after completing a fellowship at the famous Mayo Clinic in America. The story goes that Gillies encouraged him to take up plastic surgery and became his mentor. During the Second World War, 'Archie', as he was known, worked at Queen Victoria Hospital in East Grinstead, West Sussex, where he took care of Royal Air Force pilots who were badly burned during the Battle of Britain. He took on the rather remarkable mission of trying to mend these young men so that they could live normal lives. To make them whole again, a new type of surgery was needed. Although rhinoplasty, skin grafts and facial reconstruction had been practised for centuries, Gillies standardised these techniques and established the discipline that is called plastic surgery.

McIndoe's legacy lives on today. He helped found the British Association of Plastic, Reconstructive and Aesthetic Surgeons (BAPRAS). The BMI McIndoe Surgical Centre now occupies the building that once housed the burns unit, which ironically was the site of the popular UK edition of *Extreme Makeover*. What a difference 65 years make!

As long as we have wrinkles, there will always be a market for everything anti-ageing and today we are witnessing a sea change in attitudes towards cosmetic enhancement. There has been a massive growth in the sales of anti-ageing products in the UK. A survey by Alliance Boots reported that one in three women over 30 uses in the UK over anti-ageing products, and these women spend more than £650 million on them each year.

It should come as no surprise that cosmetic surgery is also growing by leaps and bounds. Figures from the British Association of Aesthetic Plastic Surgeons (BAAPS) show a rise of 35 per cent in one year. Age-reversing procedures have seen the greatest increase: a 42 per cent boost in facelifts and a 50 per cent rise in eyelid surgery. The top-ranked surgery was breast enlargement, which accounted for 20 per cent. In 2006 more than 65,000 cosmetic surgeries were carried out in the UK, costing a total of over £659 million. Most of these treatments – 89 per cent – were done on women, of course.

And that's just the beginning. Less invasive treatments such as Botox® and fillers are on offer in beauty clinics in villages all over the country. In 2005 there was a 50 per cent increase in the number of people treated with Botox®, and more than 100,000 treatments were done in the UK. It is estimated that each year over 400,000 people in Britain have non-surgical cosmetic treatments. These numbers reflect the growing acceptance of image enhancements for women (and for men too) and the obsession with cosmetic surgery that seems to be spreading across the globe. For many, having cosmetic treatments or surgery is no longer considered a moral dilemma, social embarrassment or medical risk.

AIRBRUSHING IS THE BEST COSMETIC SURGERY

The desire to improve oneself is a natural consequence of living in our image-conscious culture. Behind virtually every A-list celebrity today is a small army of stylists, dermatologists and cosmetic surgeons ready to fluff, nip and tuck anything that needs adjustment. Women in particular face increased pressure to look younger in an age when mature celebrities who still look perfect adorn magazine covers. We don't revere ageing the way other generations have in the past. In our society, looks count.

Cosmetic treatments offer many secondary physical and psychological benefits as well. The way you feel about how you look sends a signal to the world that you are either confident and content or shy and self-conscious. When you take control of something that makes you unhappy, you remove a self-imposed barrier and ultimately improve your self-esteem tremendously.

Our dissatisfaction with our looks motivates a whole list of behaviours – losing weight, buying a new wardrobe, trying a new hairstyle, changing our make-up and, in some cases, having a go at surgery. Every woman has at least one thing she secretly wants to change about her appearance and usually a whole slew of them. It could be your father's long nose, the hooded eyelids that you've had since your twenties or muffin top that creeps out over your low-riding jeans. Who would not choose distinctive and alluring over plain and ordinary? Even if you flinch at the idea of actually going under the knife yourself, you cannot argue with the fact that youth and beauty are highly coveted commodities. Debates about cosmetic surgery are rarely limited to practical considerations: they invariably involve questions of morality. Yet ultimately, cosmetic surgery offers what our culture values most: aesthetic improvement and the preservation of youthfulness and vitality.

Aging Gradually or Aging Gorgeously

17

YOU'RE SO VAIN

Looking after yourself and striving to be the best you can be should be admired. Our ideas about what is vain have changed to the extent that vanity is no longer considered a dirty word. Whereas a woman was once considered vain if she had a facial or wax once a week, nowadays the equivalent may be regular Botox® injections. For an increasing cross section of women of all ages, beauty treatments, spa therapies, injections, peelings and surgery have become a normal way of life. The argument, from a more Victorian mindset, is that tinkering with what God gave you is only for people who have a low opinion of themselves. In my experience of talking to thousands of women over the past 25 years, most women who go in for cosmetic enhancements are pretty self-confident and very switched on.

When most people (or men) think of cosmetic surgery, they tend to think of melon-sized breasts and the wind-tunnel facelifts seen on the big screen. Everyone can spot the obvious victims of overdone cosmetic surgery. Many women say they don't want to have a lift because they have never seen a good one. 'I can always tell', is a common lament. Yet the good work is virtually undetectable. Brilliantly done lifts just look as if their owners have aged well or look good for their age – and who doesn't want that?

BE PREPARED

When you watch instant makeovers, youthifying transformations and dramatic image changes on television, it all seems like a day at the beach. There are practically no bruises, precious little swelling and almost no pain, and the best part of all is that it appears to be free. On some of these shows, the participants get it all done on the dole, which may account for their delight with the entire process. If they had to max out their Switch cards, they might think differently.

Cosmetic surgery is designed to improve contours (to lift what is

Plastic Makes Perfect

loose), whereas non-surgical procedures enhance the skin's texture (smooth lines, wrinkles and scars, and reduce pigment problems and redness). The overall mission of both is to help you look as good as your own anatomy and skin texture will allow. If you expect a transformation miracle after one little surgical procedure, you are setting yourself up for a huge disappointment. Cosmetic surgery does not deliver perfection. Many factors will contribute to the result you get, some of which are not entirely under your control or the control of your doctor. The other obvious wild card is what you expect from the procedure. As unscientific as it may seem, pure luck factors into the equation. Some people just fare better than others.

Even though society now accepts and embraces cosmetic surgery, let's face it – no reasonable woman jumps into it with a happy heart. You may be excited about the after effects, and getting through it is the means to an end. Your first time can be fraught with questions, doubts, fears and uncertainties. To make it go smoothly, prepare yourself both mentally and physically.

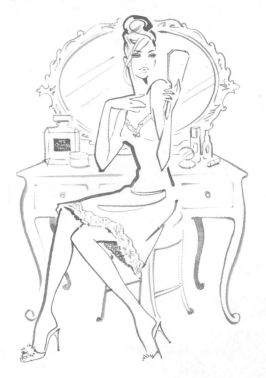

2

Tick Tock Goes Your Beauty Clock

One day you wake up, look in the mirror and realise that you are past your best. It seems like it happens that fast. The mirror is a cruel mistress. We can't stop looking in it, yet we hate to see ourselves. The cruellest of all are 9x-lighted magnifying mirrors. These seem to be getting more powerful all the time! Beyond a certain age, without your glasses you can't see what you're doing.

In the modern world, we are under intense scrutiny from all sides. Cosmetic surgeons report that business is booming since the advent of HDTV (high-density television). Every flaw is magnified on the screen, so that looking average is no longer good enough. The latest generation of laser vision surgery has taken our ability to see microscopic flaws with the naked eye towards a superhuman level. No woman over 40 wants a partner with insect-like vision!

Is it any wonder that most women start thinking about cosmetic surgery when they get depressed by what they see in the mirror? It is a terrible moment when all of a sudden you find yourself feverishly plucking out your first grey hair or having to drag up your eyelids to put on your mascara. It seems as if everything started to sag practically overnight.

WHEN SHOULD I START?

In the overall scheme of things, there is no ideal time to jump on the Botox® bandwagon. Although the trend is certainly towards doing things earlier in order to pre-empt the day when everything goes south, you can also make an argument for waiting longer, until you feel you are ready. There is no right or wrong way. Don't feel pressured into diving into the operating theatre just because all your contemporaries are already on their third lift and thirtieth peel and you feel that you have to catch up. But if everyone in your social group looks great, you won't want to feel like the older sister either. When people around you are constantly asking 'Are you tired?' or 'Are you feeling poorly?', and you aren't either, it's probably time to give cosmetic surgery some thought.

Doing it too early can be as much of a faux pas as doing it too late. In general, the best time to do surgery is when you can benefit from some intervention. Some women need a necklift in their late thirties, whereas others look tight and firm well into their fifties. It also depends on how you feel about each symptom of ageing. I have clients who baulk at the idea of a few millimetres of dangling skin, and others who aren't bothered at all by sagging, but hate their crow's feet and puffy eyelids.

Typically, botulinum toxin and fillers (all the procedures I mention here are described later in this book) can be started in your twenties and thirties. Liposuction of the neck and fatty eyebag removal may need to be done early as well, as there may be a hereditary component – if hooded eyes or goitre necks run in your family, it's hard to escape your genes. Lifting the eyes, brows and neck is more commonly done in the forties and up. But these are only very general guidelines.

For the body, no rules apply. I see college girls who want their breasts enhanced for their 21st birthday. Many women wait until they have breastfed two or three children and want to have the body they used to back again. Another way to look at it is to do things when you can afford to, both in terms of time and finances. You may have to put off having the bump on your nose reduced until you are 30, even though you have been thinking about it since you entered university.

NEVER SAY NEVER

If I had a pound for every time I've heard a flawless 26-year-old with lineless skin exclaim, 'I can't imagine why women would ever stick needles in their faces!' I could have financed my facelift fund a hundred times over. My response to these naive young girls is an emphatic 'Come and see me when you hit 35!' 'Never say never' should be your attitude when it comes to cosmetic enhancements.

On the other hand, age alone is rarely a reason to have cosmetic surgery. If you are healthy and active in your seventies, you can still have a little nip or tuck, as long as you are medically cleared. However, the results will not be as good as they would have been if you had had surgery when you were younger. Nor will they last as long, because of the age of your skin and the severity of your lines, wrinkles and sagging.

YOUR REJUVENATION ROAD MAP

Imagine a grape shrivelling up and becoming a raisin. It starts off juicy, round and smooth, and gradually becomes dull, rough and wrinkly. That's essentially the grim reality of what happens as you age. One day you look in the mirror and think to yourself, 'How did that happen?' But in fact you have been in a state of decline from the day you were born. Here's an outline of what you can expect in each decade of your life, and what you can do about it.

THE TWENTIES: THE AGE OF ESTABLISHING GOOD HABITS

You probably haven't seen any real signs of skin damage yet, unless you are a hard-core party girl. The epidermis renews itself every 28 to 30 days. What lies beneath, however, are changes that will reveal themselves when you least expect them. The stratum corneum, or the top layer of dead skin cells, becomes slightly thicker. Smokers may see the beginning of fine lines near the eyes and mouth. If you are a squinter, you may see crow's feet and even small furrows in the brow.

What should I do?

The twenties are about setting up a sturdy foundation for a lifetime of smart skincare. Women of a certain age often look back fondly on their twenties as a time when they could stay out all night and get up for work in the morning looking fresh and rested. But that does not last forever. Although more women in their twenties are looking after their skin than in my generation, the real challenge is convincing 20-year-olds that the more they abuse their skin now, the more they will pay for it later. This is the time to focus on prevention, and keeping skin clear.

The number-one anti-ageing treatment for 20-somethings is a daily dose of SPF 15. Since you haven't yet seen much evidence of sun damage, it may be tempting to skip it, but the earlier you start, the more damage you can prevent. Even the darkest skin tones need SPF to prevent blotches and discolouration. Apart from ageing wrinkles caused by sun, pre-cancers (called actinic keratoses) show in your twenties and thirties, particularly if you are fair and spend a lot of time in the sun. Some of these lesions can turn into skin cancers. Vitamin A-based products and antioxidants should be applied topically and sunscreen should be worn daily.

If acne persists into your twenties, good treatment options include photo rejuvenation, blue light or laser-like treatments using a topical medicine. Once your skin is clear, stubborn acne scars can be treated with various lasers. If your muscles are working overtime, early frown lines, forehead wrinkles and crow's feet can be stopped short by using Botox®.

> **FAUX COSMETIC SURGERY QUICK FIXES**
>
> - Push-up bra
> - Make-up lesson
> - Home microdermabrasion kit (see Chapter 12)
> - Great haircut
> - Losing a dress size

THE THIRTIES: THE AGE OF RECOGNITION

By the time you reach your thirties, you have survived the awkwardness of the teenage years and the self-discovery of your twenties and are more in sync with your body.

Your thirties are the decade when cell turnover starts to slow down. Skin can look dull and sluggish. Fibroblasts (the forerunners to collagen and elastin) get lazy, collagen and elastin start to diminish, which results in a loss of firmness, and brown spots turn up. The first hints of sun damage begin to escalate into visible changes. The lines between the nose and the mouth (nasolabial folds) deepen. Forehead furrows multiply, and tiny lines begin to sprout all over. Every time you smile, frown, raise your eyebrows, laugh or cry you can see fissures that may still be transient but will soon become permanent. The moment you spy your first wrinkle can be a humbling experience.

What should I do?

Improve on the good habits you established in your twenties. Daily SPF 15+ is a priority to keep your skin radiant and even in colour. Consistent exfoliation with light peels and microdermabrasion works wonders to keep skin clear.

If you are keen to try a more aggressive approach, consider entering the Botox® zone. Repetitive motion of muscles is part of what caused the wrinkles, and Botox® works by reducing muscle activity, literally stopping your muscles from contracting. Studies have shown that the earlier you start using it, the more you can slow down the formation of deep wrinkles. Photo-rejuvenation treatments are good for skin tone and texture.

TOP THREE PREVENTATIVE TREATMENTS

If you're keen to do something that actually slows down facial ageing, instead of just correcting the signs, this trio will go far to keep you looking fabulous for your fortieth:

- Broad-spectrum (UVA/UVB) SPF 15 or higher
- Botox®
- Intense pulsed light therapy.

THE FORTIES: WHEN IT STARTS TO HIT THE FAN

In your forties, everything hits you all at once. Pigmentation problems arise as earlier sun exposure really catches up with you. Broken and dilated capillaries increase. New lines around your eyes, forehead and mouth occupy your thoughts. You notice that the corners of your mouth tend to turn down, which can make you look sad. Wrinkles settle in for the long haul and get comfortable. Lips shrink, hips expand and nipples point to your bunions. Loss of firmness – especially around your jawline – rears its ugly head as you approach your big birthday (your fiftieth). This is the decade when the sinking and sagging begins.

What should I do?

You don't have to take it lying down (although lying down does make sagging disappear – try lying on your bed and holding a mirror above your head). Peels and intense pulsed light treatments can even out skin tone and improve texture. Botox® is brilliant for lines around the eyes, forehead and mouth. Fillers come into their own for plumping furrows and creases, and shrinking lips. For sagging, you may opt for some minimally invasive lifting and eyelid skin removal.

This is the time to tighten up your skin. Thanks to the latest crop of less-invasive treatments, such as Thermage® and ReFirme®, you can get a lifting effect without surgery. Light treatments for the hands, neck and décolleté may be indicated, as these areas will show signs of age more than the face if you have neglected them in the past.

> **TOP THREE INSTANT-REWIND TREATMENTS**
>
> - Botox® for frown lines
> - filler for nasolabial folds (nose-to-mouth lines)
> - peels to even out the skin

THE FIFTIES: IT'S ALL GOING SOUTH

In your fifties, everything that began in your forties gets more intense. Fine lines on the cheeks become deeper-etched lines. Creases from the nose to the mouth or from the corners of the mouth down deepen. Age spots cluster and darken. Your skin sheds dead cells more slowly and in clumps instead of one at a time, so you lose your radiance. Collagen breaks down and production decreases, so skin loses thickness and support structure. Sebaceous glands grow larger but produce less oil, so your skin is dryer. Melanocyte production decreases, which means you tan less evenly and burn more easily.

The oestrogen slump in the first five years post menopause weakens collagen and causes slackening. Your neck begins to get crêpey. Just as your skin loses plumpness, your hair becomes finer, too, because of low estrogen levels.

What should I do?

You may have a surplus of concerns to be addressed, including lines, wrinkles, laxity, volume loss, blotches, white spots and brown spots. In your fifties, you may need skin tightening and resurfacing treatments on a higher setting and more frequently than you needed in your forties. For fine wrinkles and coarse texture, a laser or light-based procedure can come to your rescue by stimulating the collagen remodelling process. Age spots on the face or hands from holidays in Marbella can become just memories with the help of bleaching agents, peels and lasers. Sculptra® injections can supplement your depleted collagen supply, restore volume and smooth out wrinkles and deeper nasolabial (nose-to-mouth) lines. Fillers are very important to a 50-year-old face, and deeper fillers work nicely to plump you up where you're sinking. As for the lines, Botox® is still the best choice, and resurfacing treatments offer more dramatic results for etched lines. For sagging and slackening, surgery may offer the most benefits.

THE SIXTIES: COMING TO TERMS WITH AGEING

Women in their sixties have loose, sagging skin at least somewhere and usually everywhere. It comes with the territory. Skin cells have 30 per cent less natural moisture now than when you were younger, so you are noticeably drier, thinner, tighter and flakier. Lack of moisture also contributes to slow cell turnover and repair, and a lifetime of inconsistent sun protection means that age spots show up regularly. Yellow, tan or brown discolourations are common, as are wrinkles that extend beyond the eye and mouth areas.

What should I do?

At 60, you can still be in the game, but it takes a bigger effort (and budget). I have clients who are working, vital, active women who look great and have more energy than I had at half their age. And they want to look good through their sixties and beyond. Most of the strategies for skin rejuvenation during your fifties will also work as you enter the next decade, but more slowly and to a lesser degree.

WHAT BRINGS YOU TO THE COSMETIC SURGEON'S ROOMS?

It could be something as innocuous as watching your partner get whiplash while turning to look at a shapely waitress. Catching a glimpse of yourself in a shop window as your chins are obstructing the path of the collar of your blouse can elicit shock and horror. Everyday occurrences can start your wheels turning.

The pressures of a career, finding and keeping a partner, and leading a busy, active life, all contribute to the list of reasons hordes of women seek cosmetic enhancements to bolster their self-esteem. Having it all is only half the battle; keeping it all is the hard part.

TRIGGER EVENTS

- Losing a partner
- Wanting a new partner
- Retirement
- New job
- Being made redundant
- Empty nest syndrome
- Moving house
- Big birthday (50 for a woman)
- Inheriting a bit of money
- Ex getting remarried
- Being mother of the bride
- School reunion

UNREALISTIC EXPECTATIONS

Some people fantasise that changing their bodies with cosmetic surgery will transform their lives. Some people are drawn to surgery to seek approval outside themselves. Unfortunately, it's not that simple. Most people do feel better, physically and emotionally after surgery. But if you're expecting a Cinderella-like transformation, you're heading for a let-down. Having your eyes done or your breasts enlarged is not going to save a failing marriage, give you a social life or cure deep-rooted psychological problems. People who want to change or improve a specific physical trait – such as a large nose or saddlebags – are usually more satisfied than people who go to a surgeon with the attitude of 'I don't feel attractive – fix it for me.' Cosmetic surgery is an emotional undertaking and you have to be honest with yourself.

Ultimately cosmetic surgery should be only one part of a larger self-improvement plan, rather than as a panacea for an otherwise unfulfilling life. Women who have a sense of balance, who can incorporate surgery into the bigger picture, are the most satisfied in the long run.

NIP TIP
Never have cosmetic surgery in the middle of a life crisis. You need to be calm and focused to make sensible choices and sail through the process with ease. If your agenda is to totally rebrand yourself, you will have too much riding on the outcome of any procedure to be able to keep it in proper perspective.

WHAT KIND OF PATIENT ARE YOU?

The hardest people to please are artistic or very analytical types. For example, graphic artists, painters, photographers, interior decorators, fashion designers, make-up artists, architects and anyone in a profession that requires a keen eye are generally tough critics. Their attention to detail makes them challenging to satisfy. Funnily enough, many cosmetic surgeons are artists in their own right. Another hard-to-please group is therapists and psychoanalysts – they tend to overthink the process and dwell on minutiae. Nurses, doctor's wives and doctors are also notorious for having a mishap. They are inclined to focus on what might go wrong, instead of what will go right. It can be a self-fulfilling prophecy – they think it will go wrong, so it does.

Tick Tock Goes Your Beauty Clock

29

Ask The Beauty Junkie®

What will keep my neck looking young?
Don't assume that your face stops at your chin. Use anti-ageing creams on your neck too and always wear sunscreen there. Neck skin is thin and has fewer oil glands, so it needs constant hydration. Retinols and peptides can rejuvenate the neck. Botox® is good for softening neck-muscle bands. Skin-tightening devices work on the neck as well.

What part of the face ages first?
The eyelid area tends to show visible signs of ageing because the skin is thinnest and most delicate there. (The soles of your feet have the thickest skin, in case you were curious.) Obviously, the most fragile skin is where the effects of sun, time and stress show up first. The eyelid area also gets the most movement and manipulation from squinting, rubbing, putting in contact lenses and applying eye make-up. The eyelid area can get veiny and dark from a combined assault from sun, asthma and allergies, sleep deprivation, salt intake, nutritional deficiencies and daily wear and tear. The discolouration can be related to iron pigment from red blood cells: when blood passes through the veins close to the surface of the skin it can cause a bluish tint. The more transparent your skin, the darker and more pronounced the flaws. Troughs or hollows tend to form under the eye because of fatty tissue loss. Genetics play a role too: Asian and Mediterranean skin types are more prone to dark rings around the eyes, which can be a source of aggravation.

Does running age your face faster?
The benefits of a regular exercise programme far outweigh the downsides. However, runners often look gaunt and wasted because they have very little body fat, which shows up as an ageing face. Regular jogging can loosen up the microscopic attachments that bind muscle to skin, leading to skin sagging. Lower-impact exercise like biking, swimming, elliptical machines, yoga or Pilates don't produce a jarring effect on joints and skin.

Plastic Makes Perfect

3

Your Right
to Choose

Choosing the right procedure or treatment plan for cosmetic surgery involves many individual yet related factors including what you can spend, how much time you can take off work, school or play, your pain tolerance, your acceptance of scars and the inevitable fear factor. Some procedures are not as scary as they may seem. For example, many people linger under the misconception that liposuction is a brutal operation where a surgeon savagely sticks pointy tube-like instruments made of steel into your cottage-cheese thighs and sucks out pearly yellow globs of fat. In fact, it is a fairly gentle, almost rhythmic procedure with tiny little scars and when it is done properly, it can seem that every step has been carefully choreographed by the Royal Ballet.

FINDING DR RIGHT

There is never only one 'best' doctor or surgeon for any procedure; rather there are many competent doctors who can give you an excellent result. They are located in all sorts of places from big cities such as London to the heartland of America. But you have to put some work into finding one that is right for you. Although it may be tempting, you can't just go up to a woman in Sainsbury's and ask 'Excuse me, but who is your plastic surgeon?'

Anyone with a medical degree can call himself a cosmetic surgeon, advertise the services of a cosmetic surgeon and perform them at will. There have been cases reported of pseudo-doctors masquerading as cosmetic surgeons and operating in back-alley clinics under the radar of authorities until disaster struck and resulted in a serious complication or death. So make sure your doctor has the necessary background and experience. Approach the quest to find your doctor like a woman on a mission. You can do this – it's encoded into your DNA at birth. First, you have to develop a strategy.

1. What you want and what you need

It's all about prioritising. You need a vague idea of what body part or area you want to tackle first. You can't do it all, and going on an endless mission of multiple stages will get tedious, not to mention prohibitively expensive. Start with what bothers you the most right now.

2. Where

Get out a map and think about where you would like to have a little work done. Is it Beverly Hills because they do the most lifts there? Does a private clinic in Paris appeal to you? Or is Harley Street the best because it's closer to home? Consider where you have family and friends, and if you have a second home or place where you might like to recover.

3. Who

Gently ask some of your most savvy girlfriends if they know any great doctors for lifts, lasers or whatever treatment you think you need. Get references, referrals and information on which doctors to avoid from multiple sources such as beauty experts, hair and make-up stylists, photographers, cosmetic dentists and healthcare professionals.

4. When

Take out your diary and start crossing off impossible dates and ticking anything that could work. Count backwards from the day; for example, if you have to give a presentation on 23 October, count backwards fourteen days to 9 October to find the last possible date when you can have something (small) done and still look decent. See also page 66.

5. How

The 'how' part involves a whole host of issues. How do I break it to my partner? (Get him drunk.) How can I hide it from my children? (Send them to Grandma's house.) How can I get the time off work? (Plot and plan for it in advance.) How can I find the right doctor? (Ask around, do your homework, see a few.) The answers to other such 'how' questions will become apparent as you keep reading.

Note that I deliberately left out 'why' from the five-point plan. If you are still struggling with 'why' – as in 'Why can't I just accept the way I look and get on with it?' – do a little soul searching, re-read Chapter 1 or

Your Right to Choose

have a chat with your vicar. These are personal decisions every woman must make for herself. If you are not sure, don't do it.

THE WHO

Referrals from a friend who has had cosmetic surgery can be useful. But surgery, recovery and results will vary tremendously, and the best doctor for your sister-in-law may not turn out to be your cup of tea.

Your GP may seem an obvious source, but not every GP knows who is the best for faces or who does the most breasts. GPs usually recommend a name they have heard of, or more often, someone at the local NHS hospital, who may or may not do much cosmetic surgery at all. Ask other medical specialists such as your gynaecologist or dentist for a referral. You could get lucky and get a great referral. In my experience, nurses, registrars or surgeons in training and anaesthetists know who the best surgeons are. They work right in the operating theatre – where there is no way to hide your abilities or fudge the results. What you see on the operating table is what you get.

A MATTER OF DEGREE

Deciphering medical qualifications is a minefield, especially when the country of training dictates the acronym that goes after the practitioner's name.

Ch.M. (MS, M.Ch.)	Master of Surgery
DDS	Doctor of Dental Surgery
DM.D	Doctor of Dental Medicine
DO	Doctor of Osteopathic Medicine
FACS	Fellow American College of Surgeons
FDSRCS	Fellow of Dental Surgery
FRACS	Fellow Royal Australasian College of Surgeons
FRCP	Fellow Royal College of Physicians
FRCI	Fellow Royal College of Surgeons of Ireland
FRCS (MRCS)	Fellow Royal College of Surgeons
FRCS (Plast)	Fellow Royal College of Surgeons (Plastic Surgery)

FRCSED	Fellow Royal College of Surgeons of Edinburgh
MBCh.B. (MB.BS)	Bachelor of Medicine, Bachelor of Surgery
MD	Medical Doctor
M.Sc.	Master of Science
ND	Doctor of Naturopathic Medicine
Ph.D.	Doctor of Philosophy
RGN (RSCN)	Registered General Nurse
RCNNP	Registered General Nurse Nurse Practitioner

EDUCATE YOUR GUESS

The Internet is a primary source for all things medical. However, it is loaded with a wealth of information and misinformation, often contradictory and rarely policed by any official source. There are many commercial websites that offer referrals to doctors and financing programmes, and some stoop to all sorts of gimmicks to lure patients.

Bulletin boards, bloggers and chat rooms are also not good sources of accurate tips and rock-solid recommendations. These can breed seemingly endless chains of irrelevant comments from self-proclaimed 'experts'. Anonymous postings offer zero credibility as to the IQ of their source. What makes you think that someone who calls herself 'Lipqueen628' knows any more than you do?

Adverts in the back of glossies and on the web can be misleading too. Be wary of advertisements that promise lunchtime lifts or painless liposuction, use hyped-up names for procedures and vague language to explain what they do, and offer guaranteed results. In the UK and many EU countries, individual doctors are not legally permitted to advertise that they are 'the best cosmetic surgeon' or toot their own horns. However, a clinic or hospital may advertise.

The same cosmetic surgeons are often interviewed and quoted over and over again. Media coverage on its own offers no guarantee of a doctor's qualifications. A doctor's appearance on television is neither an endorsement of his skills nor a testament to his clinical excellence. Never pick a surgeon on the basis of a glitzy website, slick advertising or media appearances alone.

Your Right to Choose

Individual doctors' websites are a good place to learn about their training and hospital affiliations, but you also need to get a sense of whether you feel comfortable with the doctor. I like to look at a doctor's face – see if there is a twinkle in his eye or if he has the stone-cold face of a serial killer. After all, this is a human relationship. You don't have to fall in love with your surgeon (though many women do), or even become friends, but you do have to feel confident that he (or she) is your guy (or gal).

BEWARE OF COSMETIC SURGERY CONSULTANTS, ADVISERS AND OTHER SELF-NAMED EXPERTS

Having a few surgeries by a handful of doctors does not an expert make. Neither does dating a cosmetic surgeon. Not all 'consultants' are independent or impartial. If a consultant 'represents' a handful of doctors or, as in some cases, just one doctor, he or she is not offering objective advice. It may be hard to determine exactly what motivates paid referral arrangements, and it is reasonable to be suspicious before signing on. If you are getting a 'free consultation', someone is being compensated along the line.

BOOK A CONSULTATION

There are some things that are non-negotiable with my clients. One of my mantras is that you *must* have at least two consultations before having anything surgical. And my consultation with them does not count as one of the two. Contrary to popular belief, I am neither a nurse nor a doctor, although I have been called both on many occasions. In fact, if you were even thinking that I am a nurse, you have lost the plot and should go back to square one! No sensible person should make assumptions about anyone's medical qualifications without looking them up, double checking or viewing a wall covered in neatly framed diplomas.

You need to have proper consultations with fully qualified medical professionals. And never be afraid to get a second (or third or fourth) opinion. The general rule is that you should see at least two surgeons before scheduling a major surgical procedure such as a

NIP TIP
Make sure the doctor you choose for your surgery is an active member of the official governing organisation of specialists. For a list of reputable specialist organisations, see page 311).

browlift or tummy tuck. For non-surgical treatments, such as a filler or intense pulse light therapy, one or two may be sufficient.

Before scheduling a consultation, request brochures describing the doctor's practice, visit websites and ring up to request materials about the procedures you are considering. Find out in advance about the range of fees so that you can ensure that you stay within your budget. Once you have narrowed down your list to a handful of suitable practitioners, schedule your consultation visits. There may be six weeks to several months' lead time to get in to a busy cosmetic surgeon, so plan accordingly. If you are keen to get in sooner, be flexible. Inform the office that if there is a last-minute cancellation, you are willing to dash in to see the doctor with very little notice.

Never go with the first or only cosmetic surgeon you see. Even if you love the first doctor you see in consultation, go to at least one or two others for confirmation and comparison. After the third, you may still find you want to go with the first one you saw, but only after you see others are you really ready to choose wisely. If it doesn't feel right, continue with the interview process.

WHAT MAKES A QUALIFIED COSMETIC SURGEON?

Take a copy of this checklist of key criteria to your consultation.

Specialises mainly in aesthetic or cosmetic surgery, NOT only breast reconstruction, paediatric deformities, burn scars or hand surgery	
Has certification by relevant medical organisations, societies, fellowships	
Has privileges at fully accredited major hospitals to perform the procedure you are considering	
Participates in continuing education in his specialty	
Has academic affiliation – a teaching hospital appointment	
Has licensed anaesthetists to administer anaesthesia	
Has a credentialled clinic staffed by experienced medical personnel	

THE CONSULTATION

The consultation is your chance to ask questions and take notes, so take a notebook and pen. Prepare a list of questions to take with you so that you don't forget anything important. You will forget most of what the surgeon tells you during the initial visit, and written notes will come in handy later on. There is no such thing as a stupid question, or asking too many questions, although surgeons are not always eager to respond to the same questions over and over again. Save any concerns about the surgeon's qualifications, training, experience and the nitty-gritty details such as fees, scheduling and payment to talk through with the nurses and secretaries, who have more time, and usually more patience. Surgeons are typically big-picture people; they don't like to fuss with the small stuff.

The initial consultation may be with a nurse, receptionist or office manager; however, your evaluation should be with the doctor who will actually be performing the procedure. Personally, I don't trust a doctor who doesn't take notes. There is no way he can remember the specifics of what you discussed without writing them down. Doctors are not superhumans, despite what they believe. They also have a short attention span.

Be wary of any doctor who strong-arms you to have a number of procedures that are unrelated to the reason for your consultation. The surgeon should not pressurise you into making any decisions on the spot, either. For example, if you came in for a breastlift, and he offers, 'I can take the bump off your nose at the same time,' that could be a warning sign that

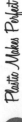

this particular doctor is too eager and aggressive. However, if you came in for your eyelids and your doctor suggests a browlift as well, he is simply doing his job. It is impossible to consult on one part of your face without at least mentioning an adjacent or related area that needs doing as well.

WHAT YOU WANT

Most cosmetic surgeons will hand you a mirror and ask you to point out what is bothering you. Be as specific as possible in communicating what you want. Be prepared to show the surgeon what you don't like about your face or body, what looks different or not as good as it used to, and what you want to change, improve or get rid of altogether. What you may innocently call your 'cheekbone' he may refer to as your 'malar eminence', so never assume you are speaking exactly the same language. Point to the area in the mirror so that you're both on the same page. The consultation process should be a team effort.

Alternatively, there is the know-it-all who walks in and states unequivocally, 'I need a mid-facelift.' Surgeons are born control freaks, and even though you might not have caught it, he has just rolled his eyes in your direction. In my experience, this is a bad approach and will backfire. Although you may think you know what you want because you know someone who had the procedure or you saw it done on television or in a magazine, it may not be right for you. Your skin type, degree of sagging, individual ability to heal, bone structure, overall health and any earlier interventions in the area will determine to some extent the quality of the result you can expect. Describe the effect you want to achieve, and be open to hearing what each surgeon recommends.

One of the most common mistakes is to zero in on one concern while missing something else that needs attention. For example, fixating only on your droopy eyelids when your brows are sinking; having your neck done but ignoring the crinkly lines around your mouth; or having only your jowls tidied up when the crease between your eyebrows looks like Moses parting the Red Sea. Changing or rejuvenating one feature on your face can make your other features look different or older by comparison. It's like painting one wall of a room: the other three will look bleak in comparison.

NIP TIP
Bring some photographs of your former self (aged 25 to 35) if you are considering an anti-ageing surgery such as eyelids or facelift. Don't arrive with pictures of Claudia Schiffer's nose, Eva Longoria's chin and Catherine Zeta-Jones's eyes in hand to illustrate what you want. They are surgeons – not magicians!

British women tend to want a very natural look so that no one knows they have had any surgery. While this strategy sounds great in theory, in reality, it may land you back in the cosmetic surgeon's rooms one or two years later with sagging and puffiness you didn't expect to see again so soon. You will be devastated when faced with another £10,000 bill for round two, not to mention the fact that you will hardly be happy to go through the whole thing again – including doctor's visits, medical tests, photographs, bruising, swelling, time out of your life and the risk of being outed by a meddling friend.

My best advice is to do surgery properly, and make sure it will last. To have a surgical lift of the face or body and end up with floppy chins or a saggy tummy before you turn around will be very disappointing. A lift that is too conservative is a bit like Chinese food – two hours later you're hungry again.

Doctors don't always realise what a big deal surgery is for women, that we have a lot riding on the outcome. When it goes wrong, or turns out less than satisfactory, women go through a whole spectrum of emotions – guilt, blame, shame, anger, regret and embarrassment. Bad cosmetic surgery is far far worse than ageing or living with the hand you were dealt (small breasts, thin lips, thunder thighs, etc). It calls more attention to itself.

MEDICAL QUESTIONS

For a proper consultation with a cosmetic surgeon, you need to dig a bit deeper into his level of training and qualifications, and how he performs the treatment(s) recommended for you. Ask about the basics of the procedure and how they apply to you specifically. After a consultation for a facelift, for example, you should know exactly where the incisions will be. Understanding what the procedure can and cannot do, as well as the limitations, is quite important, in order to avoid any disappointment.

I never cease to be amazed by the lack of communication between doctors and their patients. It is usually the fault of both parties rather than one or the other. If you don't ask the right questions, you won't get the answers you need. If you don't listen carefully or the doctor doesn't make himself clear you will linger under all sorts of misconceptions.

Your doctor should fully explain the risks of the procedure – this falls under the realm of what is called 'informed consent'. If not, then his staff should clearly explain what is involved. These are the obvious issues to be covered:

- How many incisions will I have and where will they be?
- What kind of anaesthetic will be given and who will administer it?
- At which hospital will my surgery be performed?
- How long will the procedure take?
- How long are the results expected to last? (Ask for a range of months to years.)
- What is the extent of the recovery, overall healing time and time off work needed?
- What are the potential complications and side-effects associated with the procedure?
- Ask to see pre- and post-op photographs of other people the doctor has worked on, so as to see his aesthetic skills and what you can expect. If a doctor refuses to show you any, it is a great leap of faith to put your face, nose or breasts in his hands. The quality of the results a doctor can achieve is his most vital calling card. All cases are different and photos can be

RED FLAGS

Carry on looking for a cosmetic surgeon if the one you consult with:
- is unwilling to answer your questions directly
- does not explain things fully
- is impatient and irritable
- doesn't make you feel comfortable
- has an unprofessional or incompetent office staff
- pressures you into adding extra procedures you didn't ask for
- offers to squeeze you in if you pay right away

retouched or altered. Make sure he is showing you his own results and not something he just pulled off the Internet. There is no guarantee that your results will be the same.

Finally, ask yourself how you felt after the consultation. The level of communication with your physician and his staff, as well as the confidence he inspires in you, will be vital to the success of your surgery. At the end of the day, you have to go with your gut feeling. If after your consultation you have a queasy feeling in the pit of your stomach, the doctor is probably not the one for you. Go with your gut instincts – they are usually spot on.

Alexandra's débâcle

After seeing three cosmetic surgeons she had found in her local paper, Alexandra, aged 28, was in a terrible quandary. She wanted something subtle to refresh her looks, but nothing too drastic. The first doctor suggested cheek and breast implants, although Alexandra clearly said that she didn't want to change her face and never even mentioned her breasts. The second doctor told her he would use a laser to smooth out her wrinkles (she didn't think she had any yet) and plump up her nose-to-mouth lines with a filler – but didn't tell her which one he would use. The last doctor she saw told her she needed the fat removed from under her eyes and a new chin. All this sounded way more than what Alexandra was up for, and she was put off. When she came to see me, we talked through her goals and budget. Implants of any kind were off the table – she didn't want anything made bigger. She had lovely skin with the odd spot or two and the mere hint of crow's feet. I referred her to a cosmetic doctor who suggested that all she needed was a bit of Botox® around the eyes, and he gave her an anti-acne skincare regime. Alexandra was happy with that. Her treatment ended up costing £400 instead of the £4,000 and up she had been quoted by the clinics she had been to.

Once you have zeroed in on two or three doctors, you can go back to see the frontrunners again to make the final cut.

When it comes to surgery, choosing a doctor is the most important decision you will make. There is no substitute for expertise and skills. You get what you pay for. Go with the best doctor you can afford – which means not necessarily the most expensive but the most experienced and qualified person to do the procedure you are considering. You should arrive at the conclusion that this is the best doctor for you on the basis of considerable research and confirmation from more than one source as well as a little bit of woman's intuition.

NIP TIP
Make sure that the surgeon with whom you had your consultation actually performs your surgery. An operating room technician or nursing staff may assist, but the procedure should be conducted by the surgeon you chose. Do not allow your surgeon to be substituted at the last minute – they are not interchangeable. Insist on having the surgeon to whom you wrote your cheque!

When you have settled on a doctor and you are ready to go ahead, you can schedule your procedure. There may be a longer wait for surgery than for a consultation. Busy cosmetic surgeons are booked well in advance, so plan accordingly. You want to eat at the restaurant that has the most cars (preferably Jaguars) in the car park. The same goes for a cosmetic surgeon.

Try to see the doctor who will perform your procedure once more before the operation. The next visit should be scheduled closer to the date of surgery so that you have another opportunity to ask last-minute questions and clarify everything. You may still have some sleepless nights and pre-surgery jitters, but by the second meeting you should feel good about the doctor you have chosen. If you do not, then have another think about it.

WHEN SURGERY IS NOT THE ANSWER

There are occasionally times when a surgeon will refuse to operate on a patient.

Our nip-and-tuck culture has produced some extreme cases. There are a growing number of people, especially young women, who suffer from body dysmorphic disorder (BDD), also known as 'imagined ugliness syndrome'. They become so convinced that they are unattractive that no amount of surgical enhancement will satisfy their desire to

Your Right to Choose

change their bodies. BDD is said to affect 7–12 per cent of cosmetic surgery patients (men and women equally). Psychologists consider it to be an obsession with a physical flaw to such a point that it interferes with day-to-day functioning.

BDD sufferers express distorted ideas about their body and can become preoccupied with an imagined defect. A relatively unnoticeable flaw, such as a tiny scar or a slightly raised mole, can cause significant concern, impairing their ability to deal with life. They tend to avoid social situations just because they feel too ugly to be seen or are convinced that everyone will stare at them. They compulsively try to hide the offending feature with clothing or gestures. They may become recluses – 'I can't go out of the house looking like this.' Or they may constantly stare in the mirror and point to what is bothering them – 'Can't you see it? It's right there!'

Coming into a clinic with images of celebrities the patient wants to look like, requesting multiple consultations with endless questions and having repeat procedures are warning signs to cosmetic surgeons that the patient may be suffering from BDD.

> **BDD**
>
> The clinical test for BDD (body dysmorphic disorder) is whether the perceived flaw can be seen at a normal conversational distance. If it can't, it's not significant.

In cases of BDD, cosmetic surgery will not get to the root cause of the problem because physical flaws are not the real issue. The disorder starts with how the sufferer feels about him- or herself. BDD is usually treated with antidepressants and intensive psychotherapy.

Many cosmetic surgeons try to screen their patients for emotional stability, but it is sometimes hard to detect after one brief meeting. Regrettably, more doctors today can be persuaded to operate on someone who thinks cosmetic surgery will change her life. It takes courage and conviction to recommend to a prospective (paying) patient that she seek intervention from a therapist, psychologist or psychiatrist. Some surgeons may think, 'If she wants it, why shouldn't I do it for her?' But the surgeon can choose not to do it, and he may be doing the patient a favour.

Olivia's slippery slope

Olivia was a shy girl who wanted her breasts made larger in a big way. She was entering university soon and convinced her mother that having implants would give her the confidence boost she needed to fit in. Her mum struggled with this decision; no one in their family had ever done anything like this before and the operation would cost a lot of money. Olivia prevailed and her implants were a graduation present. For her first two terms, she loved her breasts, was happy at college and had a boyfriend. But when she came home for the summer holiday, she had a new obsession. Convinced that her boyfriend was cheating on her because her body wasn't up to scratch, she was now focused on having her bottom lifted. Her mum saw Olivia as a striking young woman with a lovely face and figure, but Olivia still didn't feel good about herself. Fortunately, the plastic surgeon who did her breasts agreed with Olivia's mum and refused to operate on her again.

PAY DAY

Cosmetic surgery is a luxury service, and it can be expensive. Fees for cosmetic surgery vary widely, depending on the extent of the procedure, the number of procedures being done, the amount of time it will take to perform, where you are having it done – as you would expect, fees tend to be higher in central London than in Newcastle – and, of course, the surgeon. Most non-invasive procedures start in the hundreds and rise to the thousands pretty quickly. Surgery starts in the neighbourhood of £3,000 and can get up to the sticker price of a Mercedes before you know it. And all fees are expected to be paid in advance – with cash or plastic.

Most doctors accept personal cheques, cash and major credit cards. Some clinics also participate in financing programmes to help you pay the costs over time. If you don't have the money, personal loans are very tempting. In most cases, I discourage my clients from going down this path. It works well for the clinic because they get your money up

NIP TIP
There is no such thing as cheap plastic – you get what you pay for. In fact, cheap plastic can end up costing twice (or three times) the price you paid. If you are not happy with the results, it can cost a fortune to have it redone.

Your Right to Choose

45

front, but you are faced with paying off the price of your rhinoplasty or liposuction for the next couple of years at staggering interest rates (often 18–25 per cent). If you go into debt to finance breast implants, what happens if they don't give you what you were hoping for? If you're not happy with the outcome of your surgery, when the bill is due it will be a constant reminder of your experience. If you cannot afford to write a cheque for the procedure, or put it on your MasterCard and pay it off quickly, save up and wait until you can.

Never choose a doctor for a cosmetic procedure solely on the basis of cost. While the surgical fee needs to be considered, it should not be the primary factor in selecting a plastic surgeon. Take on board that the surgeon's training, certification and experience are keys to the success of cosmetic surgery.

HIDDEN COSTS

When deciding to have cosmetic surgery, it may seem logical to add something else, since you're going under anyway. Certainly, doing a few procedures in one stage (for example, a facelift and eyelids, or a tummy tuck and lipo on your thighs) makes good economical sense and saves you from having another round of time out of work at a later date. But there is a limit to how many procedures and how much anaesthesic you can safely have at once – no one can have a total head-to-toe surgical makeover in an afternoon! And further procedures can add to your costs and to your recovery.

Most doctors charge a consultation fee that is paid on the day. Consultation fees range from £25 to £200. In some cases, this fee may be added to the cost of the procedure you are having. A consultation with a nurse or clinic manager may be free, but as I said earlier you should insist on seeing the surgeon who will actually be doing the work before scheduling. Then there is a fee for the doctor doing the procedure. Additional costs include your hospital stay and an anaesthetist, which may be a fixed amount or one based on the number of hours the surgery takes. Hospital fees in the UK can be a real shocker; they can be almost as high as the surgeon's fee. Ask for a breakdown so that you understand all the costs involved in advance. Like renovating a house, surgery will always cost more than you anticipated.

WHAT HAPPENS IF I GET COLD FEET?

Many doctors will require a non-refundable deposit in order to hold a surgical date, which can vary from a nominal amount to 10–25 per cent or more of the total fee. The balance of the fee is usually due two to four weeks prior to your surgery date. If you cancel surgery without adequate notice, many doctors will charge a cancellation fee or retain your deposit or the entire fee.

TRAVELLING ABROAD FOR SURGERY

The world is indeed a smaller place today. Travelling out of your home town or country for surgery is on the rise. The concept of travelling a few hours by plane in search of a really great lift, a unique doctor who offers something you can't get at home, total privacy, better aftercare or just to get away from the distractions of your daily life certainly appeals to many.

At first glance, travelling out of the country for cosmetic surgery may seem glamorous and exciting. However, it is not always practical or safe. You need a complete medical and a proper comprehensive consultation with the surgeon who will have your face or body in his hands. You can't just arrive after a long-haul flight and jump into the operating theatre in a foreign country.

Evaluating the training and credentials of doctors abroad is a minefield. Qualifications vary from country to country, and there is no single international governing body that regulates standards for quality, training and safety. Don't just accept the medical qualifications of doctors at face value without doing some research. 'Trained in America' could translate into attending a two-hour course in Cleveland five years ago and is not a guarantee of anything.

Many offshore clinics are not operated or owned by doctors, so the standards of care may not be up to snuff. Beware of travel agents or representatives who handle all your arrangements in lieu of a proper consultation with the surgeon who will be performing your surgery. Photographs on websites and glossy brochures may also be very misleading. In reality the theatre and recovery rooms may not look exactly as you anticipated. It is not easy to hunt for accreditations or safety standards for equipment, medical staff and emergency procedures. Many facilities located outside the UK may fail to meet minimum safety standards and operate with antiquated machines and devices. Find out if the hospital or clinic is registered with the local health authority, and if it is a fully licensed facility.

Be sure not to overlook the issue of aftercare. Determine where you will be staying after surgery, and who will be caring for you. Plan to stay in the area where you had your surgery for about a week after small procedures (eyelid surgery, breastlift, liposuction) and two weeks for anything major (face- and browlift, tummy tuck, bodylift), depending on how long the flight home will be.

You will need to be seen by your surgeon at various intervals following the operation. Flying to Capetown for a follow-up after your breast reduction is not all that simple. If you decide to have surgery away from home, ask if your surgeon has a colleague closer to the UK or where you live who could see you for follow-up care if needed. Nor are post-surgical problems easily handled if your surgeon or his nursing staff are not accessible to you. Most doctors will not be eager to handle post-op complications if they did not perform the original procedure. They will be especially reluctant if you have gone abroad to have it done in the first place. If you run into trouble, you may be left to fend for yourself or end up in the nearest A&E.

If you are planning to travel to another city, pick a place where you have a friend or relative, or bring someone along. I never recommend going off to a strange place all alone. Having someone by your side can make all the difference, even if you have chosen a first-class facility and surgeon. The language barrier is also a consideration. The doctor may speak English well enough for you to communicate, but the other medical staff may know no English at all. If you don't speak the language, have important phrases translated in advance, such as 'My face/tummy/eye hurts a lot,' and 'I'm allergic to codeine and penicillin.'

You may have no recourse if a procedure goes wrong in another country. If the doctor has no assets in the UK, you will be pretty much out of luck. In the event of a complication or the need for a revision, you will have to pay out of your own pocket.

Don't pick a tropical clinic with palm trees swaying in the ocean breeze as a place to go under the knife. It may sound enticing, but the reality of having offshore surgery is not always pretty. After surgery, you won't be up for safaris or sunbathing. Bed rest is standard post-operative procedure; golf, tennis, horseback riding and swimming are verboten. Lounging around the pool is also a big no-no. You will be covered in sunblock, sunglasses and a broad-brimmed hat. While the kids can enjoy the pool and other resort activities, you're going to be packed in ice, swathed in bandages and in hiding.

If you want a holiday, go for it without having surgery as well. But if you want to have a surgical procedure done properly, pick a highly qualified surgeon regardless of location.

There is no such thing as cheap plastic – you get what you pay for. In fact, cheap plastic can end up costing twice or three times the original price. If you are not happy with the results, it can cost a fortune to have it redone.

Paula and the pina coladas

Paula's dream of a tummy tuck involved having the surgery far away from her partner and three small children, and without the worry of everyone in her little village in Somerset hearing about it. She booked herself into a clinic she found online with a charming little surgery suite and a friendly-faced doctor. When she got there, she went to the nearest tropical bar and ordered several tall pina coladas with umbrellas swirling in the glass to calm her nerves, forgetting that she was having a general anaesthetic the next morning, which was less than six hours away. Her surgery had to be postponed until the rum in her system was fully digested.

If you are keen to venture out of the UK for surgery, there are many sensible places to consider. Perhaps the number-one destination from the UK has historically been South Africa. Canada and Australia are also UK-friendly destinations, but none too close.

Europe is the obvious first choice because of proximity. My top picks based on the quality of the surgeons and facilities include France, Spain, Italy, Germany and Switzerland. America is the other way to go, with New York and South Florida topping the list because they are East Coast cities. Southern California has no shortage of great cosmetic surgeons in all price ranges, with Beverly Hills being the most expensive place to have anything done in the free world. Many Brits will make the 13-hour flight. Los Angeles caters to people from all over the world, and has first-class aftercare facilities; more men have procedures done here than anywhere else, apart from Rio.

DESTINATION NIP TUCK: A TRAVELLER'S GUIDE

Argentina Cosmetic surgery is a national pastime in Buenos Aires and the surgery vacation industry is supported by the government. Cosmetic procedures are widely available at heavily discounted prices due to the devalued currency.

Benelux Fees in Belgium and the Netherlands are extremely good value, and there are many qualified surgeons who speak perfect English, French and German. Beware of mass-market clinics that advertise heavily and seek out a reputable surgeon.

Brazil Where the cosmetic surgery craze was born; over 5,000 plastic surgeons around this sprawling country as many as in the USA. The Brazilians are world-class surgeons and are masters at making a woman 50 look 25. With 3,000 miles of beaches, their bodywork is the best to be found.

Capetown Favourable exchange rates, gorgeous scenery and qualified surgeons make this the number one destination for British women in men in search of surgery holidays, and the industry is well established here. Johannesburg is not as desirable because of the higher crime rate.

Costa Rica What South Africa is to Europe, Costa Rica is to the States. There are several qualified American-trained surgeons operating clinics and they recruit patients from Miami.

Cyprus It may be sunny, but make sure you are going to a qualified surgeon and a clinic with proper aftercare facilities.

Greece A short flight, with some nicely done clinics offering good value for money, with a warm and welcoming attitude.

India Very hi-tech with modern equipment and good nursing care, India is a relative newcomer to medical tourism but is fast becoming a big player in this new industry. English-speaking and 400 plastic surgeons.

Mexico The new Brazil, but closer to the States, and there are many good surgeons to choose from. Beware of package deals and surgery vacations that have produced some very poor results. Some Americans are going to Mexico to have weight-reduction surgeries, which are much cheaper, and offered to anyone with a few stone to lose.

Poland, Hungary, Czech Republic A growing destination for cut rate cosmetic surgery and dentistry, and fees can be as low as £1,000 for an eyelid procedure. Check out the doctor before making the trip.

South Korea Has become the Asian destination for cut-rate cosmetic operations, which are much cheaper than in Japan. Nose, cheek, chin and eye procedures are being done in South Korea in record numbers. There are reportedly about as many plastic surgeons in Korea as there are in California

Sweden Superb medical care and English-speaking nursing staff and surgeons; good value.

Sydney Although Sydney has the most surgeons, Melbourne and Perth are also popular travel destinations for surgery seekers from the UK, particularly due to the sunshine and of course, the ease of speaking the same language.

Thailand Known as the land of sex-change operations, but with the drawback of substantial HIV/AIDS problem, Thailand is emerging as a destination for medical tourism with new clinics and cheap labour to work in them.

Toronto A lovely city to have something done, perhaps not in winter though, with many conservative and qualified surgeons offering the natural look that British women seek. Montreal is also good, but further away. Vancouver is superb as well, but most people are not keen to make the longer flight.

OFF SHORE AND OFF LIMITS

The exploding cost of private health care in the UK has driven many British women to travel abroad for treatment at a fraction of the cost. Several countries, hungry for Euros and pounds, are waging an aggressive marketing campaign to attract Europeans seeking low-cost cosmetic surgery. In recent years, more countries have caught on that cosmetic surgery packages are a good source of revenue. For example, Malaysia, Thailand, Philippines and Eastern Europe are experiencing a growth spurt in clinics marketing themselves to Europeans and Americans. These countries have a long list of heavily marketed, questionable clinics offering no-frills surgery. It is not to say that all cosmetic surgeons in any one of these destinations are to be avoided. But pulling a clinic off the web is surely not sufficient reason to get on the next plane.

I urge caution when considering a place that is not exactly known for aesthetic excellence. The political, social and economic climate should be taken into consideration. In some countries, tourists are at risk of kidnap. One of my clients was planning to take her husband to Thailand for hair transplants (not through my recommendation) on the eve of the latest coup!

Dental work is the most popular procedure people have sought overseas. There are inherent risks when you are turning over your face or your body to the lowest bidder. Some patients end up happy, some are disappointed. For those who are not satisfied, they may find there is little recourse. What if you have a serious complication and you're thousands of miles from home?

Plastic Makes Perfect

Ask The Beauty Junkie®

How long are the waiting lists for cosmetic surgeons?
That depends on how busy the surgeon is, where he is located and the time of year. A typical wait may be several weeks to several months. If you can be flexible with your schedule, there is the chance of being squeezed in when there is a cancellation. It is always worth waiting for the right surgeon for you.

Can I get cosmetic surgery on the NHS?
Cosmetic surgery is considered elective, and as such is not covered on the NHS. The possible exception might be gigantic breast reductions, which could fall under the realm of reconstructive surgery – but only if your breasts are so large that they are nearly crippling you and there are serious health risks. Be prepared to queue up for 18–24 months in many areas around the country.

What can I do if something goes wrong?
Most cosmetic surgery is not completely reversible. Fortunately, though, most things can be improved, at least to some degree. Inquire about the doctor's policy on additional surgery or revisions before you have surgery. If you are not entirely satisfied with your result, find out what options you have and what can be done. If your doctor stands behind his work, he may be willing to do a revision at no additional charge or at a lesser charge within a certain amount of time, such as six months to a year. You may have to pay for the hospital and anaesthetist if required.

Will my private health insurance cover me if I have surgery abroad?
Most health insurance providers will not cover elective procedures; nor will they cover treatment outside your own country. Therefore, if you need follow-up care back home, you may have to be treated on the NHS or privately at your own expense.

4

Playing it Safe

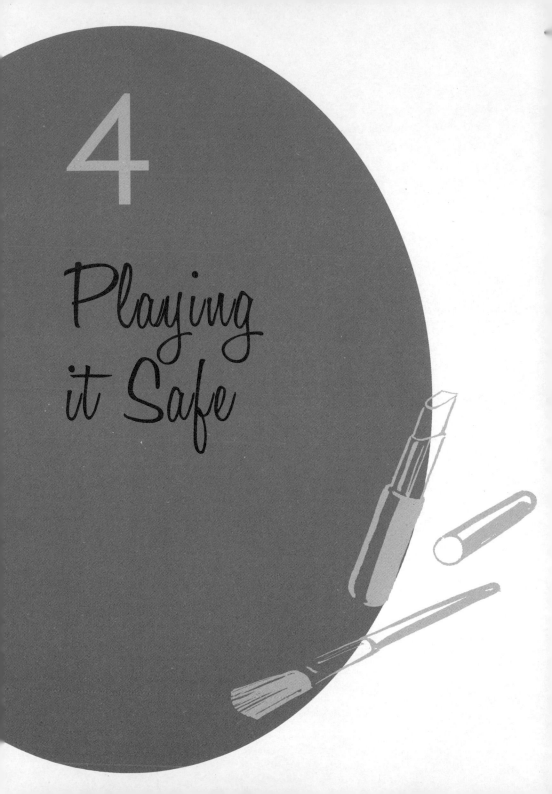

W henever a surgeon picks up a scalpel, it is real surgery, even if it is intended to beautify instead of cure disease or repair injury. Your safety is paramount. It is never worth taking unnecessary risks with your health purely for the sake of having less fat on your thighs or cartilage in your nose. It is also important to be aware of the issues that will affect your safety during surgery and a successful outcome. Real surgery should be undertaken with a high degree of seriousness, rather than the casual attitude of having a haircut or manicure. Hair and nails grow back.

WHAT TESTS ARE REQUIRED BEFORE HAVING SURGERY?

Before having surgery, you will need a medical screen for any conditions that potentially need to be dealt with before surgery. These include anaemia, clotting problems, hepatitis B or C, liver problems, diabetes, heart disease and high blood pressure. This test can be performed by your GP or at the hospital where your surgery will take place. If you are over 40, an ECG (electrocardiogram) is usually required. For women of child-bearing age, a pregnancy test may be requested. A chest X-ray may be needed as well, especially for smokers.

If you have any other medical conditions, additional testing may be requested. Ideally, you should be in optimal health before having surgery. If you have a cold or respiratory infection just before your operation, your surgery may have to be postponed. If you are running a temperature, your surgery may be postponed.

SUPERBUGS

The bacteria MRSA (methicillin-resistant *Staphylococcus aureus*) is dangerous because it is resistant to certain antibiotics and can trigger

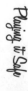

55

potentially deadly infections. It is possible to become infected with MRSA both in and out of a hospital setting. The best defence against it is good hygiene.

Most MRSA infections show up as skin infections, such as a boil or abscess that may look like a spider bite. These can be red, swollen and painful and may have pus, and most commonly show up in open wounds, mucous membranes or moist places such as under the arms. Even after the wound has healed, anyone who has been infected with MRSA may be able to transmit bacteria for months or even years.

Some doctors in the UK believe that MRSA has entered almost every public health facility in the country. The culprit is lack of cleanliness. Hospital staff are supposed to take measures to prevent the spread of MRSA and other similar superbugs, such as careful cleaning, frequent hand washing and wearing gloves when coming into contact with bodily fluids. It seems hard to imagine that any health-care worker would have to be reminded to decontaminate visibly blood-tinged surfaces, stained flooring and dirty bathroom fixtures. After all, the very purpose of a hospital is to cure and prevent disease, not to spread it. Nevertheless, superbugs exist in hospitals all over the world to some degree.

Unfortunately, there isn't much you can do to protect yourself from being infected by superbugs, short of being diligent about cleaning and washing. But when you are swathed in bandages and coming out of the anaesthetic, you can't be expected to muster the strength to change your own bed linen. Consider hiring a private nurse or having a family member at your bedside to stand guard.

THE INS AND OUTS OF ANAESTHETICS

Anaesthestics are safer now than they used to be because there are faster-acting drugs that wear off more quickly after surgery and monitoring equipment has vastly improved. Fortunately, methods of blocking pain in specific areas have advanced so much in recent years that many minor cosmetic procedures can be done using a form of a local anaesthetic. However, in the UK, most cosmetic surgeries are still performed under a general anaesthetic. The sad fact is that most of the deaths you have heard about following cosmetic surgery are related to complications from the anaesthetic, rather than the surgery itself. The good news is that complications from anaesthetics have declined dramatically, and estimates for the number of deaths attributed to anaesthesia are about 1 in 250,000.

LOCAL ANAESTHETIC

Local anaesthetic agents temporarily prevent the nerves from carrying pain messages to the brain. Local anaesthetic numbs only a part of the body, such as the hand or the nose, leaving you completely awake. The injection may be given directly into the area to be operated on or around the main trunks of the nerves that carry sensation. It may also be given as a topical spray, gel or cream applied for 30 to 60 minutes before treatment. An anaesthetist is not required.

Procedures

Fillers, lip enhancements, non-ablative laser resurfacing, fat transfer, hair restoration.

TWILIGHT ANAESTHETIC

Monitored anaesthesic, sometimes called conscious sedation, sedation analgesia or twilight sleep, is widely used for smaller cosmetic surgeries. You are conscious, but in a sleepy state and feeling no pain, and unable to respond to questions the anaesthetist asks.

Procedures

Small liposuctions, eyelid surgery, browlifts, nasal surgery, deep laser resurfacing.

GENERAL ANAESTHETIC

A general anaesthetic puts you to sleep. It is administered by injection, gas or a combination of both and causes a total loss of consciousness and sensation. Other drugs are used to take away all sensations, to relax your muscles and to keep you from going into shock.

Procedures

Tummy tuck, breast augmentation, breast reduction, bodylifts, nasal surgery, facelifts.

POSSIBLE RISKS AND SIDE-EFFECTS

Surgery is a serious business, and there is always a possibility that something will go awry. No absolute guarantees can be given. Your doctor should explain the procedure, risks, alternatives and potential complications in detail so that you know what could go wrong.

Risks can be divided into those that occur after all (or most) operations and those that are unique to a specific technique or procedure. The most common risks of cosmetic procedures include bleeding, infection and reaction to anaesthesia (such as allergies, hives, rash, vomiting and breathing difficulties). General complications from any kind of surgery include haematoma, which is a blood clot; seroma or collection of clear fluid; nerve damage; and scar tissue formation.

MOST COMMON RISKS OF COSMETIC PROCEDURES

General risks
- haematoma (blood clot)
- seroma (collection of fluid)
- skin sloughing (skin loss)
- nerve damage (temporary injury to a nerve)
- infection
- bleeding
- delayed healing
- poor scarring (raised or thickened scars)
- prolonged numbness
- reaction to anaesthetics or medications (allergic reaction, nausea, vomiting)

Serious complications
- pulmonary embolus (blood clot)
- fat embolus
- permanent nerve damage
- hypothermia
- arrhythmia (irregular heartbeat)
- aepsis (bacterial infection in the bloodstream)
- ataph infection
- perforated bowel (from liposuction)
- death (very rare!)

SMOKING GUN

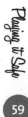

Most cosmetic surgeons will request (or even demand) that you stop smoking for two or three weeks prior to surgery. Nicotine constricts the blood vessels, and causes excessive bleeding and nasty healing problems. In some cases, smokers can actually lose a chunk of skin because of decreased oxygen flow to the skin caused by carbon monoxide. You can reduce the risks of surgery if you stop smoking beforehand and wait until you are completely healed before starting again, or preferably, quit smoking entirely. Cheating is a bad idea because you will only be cheating yourself. If you absolutely cannot quit, taper off slowly and limit yourself to as few cigarettes per day as possible. This should be your plan of last resort, because you may still have nicotine in your bloodstream at the time of surgery. Please don't lie to your doctor – ever! You're on the same team.

All forms of nicotine substitutes, including patches, gum and inhalers, simply offer an alternative source of nicotine to cigarettes. Therefore they too can increase the risk of poor healing, skin loss, scabbing, crusting and scarring. Zyban® (also known as Wellbutrin®) is a non-nicotine substitute that works at the neurological level, reducing nicotine cravings. Typically, Zyban® therapy is long term (5 to 12 weeks). Ask your doctor if it could help in your case. Hypnotherapy can also help you quit. To locate a registered hypnotherapist, see www.aphp.co.uk, www.bsch.org.uk.

Think about it this way: the more you smoke, the less tightly the surgeon can pull and the shorter amount of time your results will last. That should be a good deterrent.

Smoking in the bathroom
Gwen, the high-profile president of a cosmetics company, was frequently photographed close up and often spoke in front of large groups. She was very self-conscious about her double chin and the deep wrinkles around her mouth. She decided to have a facelift, fat injections to her smoker's lines and a chemical peel. Taking time off was the kicker – she couldn't get away from the office for more than a week. Being a chain smoker for 20 years made her situation even worse. Gwen went to a hypnotist to help her quit. At first, the treatments worked, and she lost interest in smoking. But closer to the day of her surgery, the cravings came back and she gave in. In the hospital the morning after surgery, she was caught, red handed by the head nurse, lighting up in the bathroom of her private room. Her surgeon insisted that she have round-the-clock nurses

for the next few days to make sure she did not sneak any more cigarettes. By day seven, Gwen was in no shape to show up at the office and had to work from home for another week. Her nicotine habit had caused more red and purple patches and slowed down her recovery. By day 15, Gwen looked good and was ready to once again rule her cosmetics empire, full speed ahead.

TIME HEALS ALL

When you are not happy with the results of cosmetic surgery, the natural impulse is to run kicking and screaming to the doctor, or worse, slip into a depression and refuse to leave the house. Neither of these methods are good solutions. The best way to deal with your dissatisfaction is to remain calm, rational and reasonable. Many little lumps and bumps are a perfectly normal part of the healing process and will go away on their own. The body takes time to heal itself, although every day will seem like a month to the person going through it.

1. Wait a sufficient amount of time before doing anything (at least three months).
2. Make a list of all the things you are not happy with and divide the items into 'Temporary' (swelling, bruising, numbness) and 'Permanent' (scars, shape, size).
3. Keep track of your list at specific intervals (every four to six weeks) and cross off each item as it resolves – you will be surprised at how many of these little things will fade away with time.
4. Go back to see your surgeon with your edited list (in priority order) and discuss each item.
5. Work as a team with your doctor to find a resolution, which could be to wait and see, or medical intervention or in the worst-case scenario, to have more surgery to correct the problem.
6. Before having a secondary surgery, seek out a second opinion from an impartial doctor, not related to or friends with the original surgeon (at a different hospital, city, county).

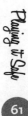

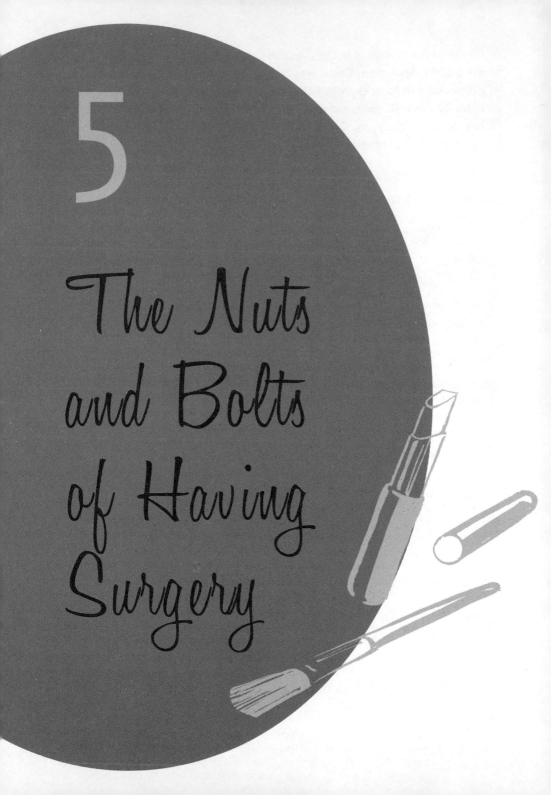

5

The Nuts
and Bolts
of Having
Surgery

FINDING THE TIME AND MONEY

The most difficult aspect of cosmetic surgery is finding the time and the money. If you really want to do it, you can probably figure out a way to save up the funds by foregoing a holiday or passing up a few shoe sales. I have clients who start what they jokingly call their 'facelift fund' wherein they squirrel away every extra penny they can.

Scheduling surgery is usually the trickiest part. Most women have to consider their husbands, lovers, children, parents, bosses, and work and travel commitments. Add to that the fact that some of the top surgeons are booked six months in advance, and picking a date to have something done can become a nightmare.

I am frequently asked about what time of year is the best to have surgery. There is no ideal season or month to undergo a cosmetic operation or treatment. This will vary depending on your lifestyle, job, family commitments and personal preferences. It may be wiser to do facial procedures at a time when you can keep a low profile. Body procedures such as liposuction and breastlifts require less time out of your life because you can hide your body better than you can conceal bruises around your eyes or neck. Surgery while your children are away at school has some advantages. If your schedule slows down during the summer, the neighbours go on holiday and the children are off school, you might find it easier to have a little work done in private. Or find out when your husband or partner will be on a business trip and steal some quiet time for yourself then.

No matter how carefully you work it out, even down to the last detail, life has a way of throwing a curve into even the best-laid plans. An event or commitment may arise at the last minute, especially if you are scheduling surgery well in advance. You may have to miss out on something: a ski trip, your best friend's son's wedding, a family reunion or the social event of the season. If that was your only window of time, you may have to wait another year. The most workable plan is often just to bite the bullet, pick a date that seems to make sense and hope for the best.

In the UK, the colder months may seem a 'more sensible' choice. It is easier to hide away and cover up with cashmere scarves and hats during January or February than it is in the hot days of July. If you plan to have any laser work, summertime may not be practical as it is hard to stay out of the sun.

If you absolutely have to look gorgeous for an upcoming event, give yourself the longest possible time to heal so that you can look and feel great in time. A minimum of three weeks for smaller things, and preferably six or more weeks for larger procedures, is advised. The woman who has a major event to host soon after surgery always seems to take the longest to heal. There is absolutely no guarantee or actionable contract that your doctor can sign as a promise that you will look 'great', 'good' or even just 'fine' by any specific date.

Surgeons are notorious for underestimating and downplaying surgery and recovery times. They are not always being dishonest, although that certainly happens; they simply do not get it. For example, there is virtually nothing that really takes 'ten minutes', and stating with confidence that 'you can go back to work after a long weekend' is rarely the case. When you really need to know, ask a woman. Nurses are usually more 'with it', and medical aestheticians know the truth because they are called on to cover up the bruising when it doesn't go away as promised.

NIP TIP
For extra-nervous girls, try not to plan too far ahead so as to avoid giving yourself too much time to think about it, worry endlessly and cancel.

NIP TIP
Assume you are going to be at the tail end of whatever range you are given and add three days for good measure in order to give yourself a cushion. So, if you are told that your bruises and swelling will go away in 5 to 10 days, assume that it will be 13 days.

Don't listen to the surgery guru in your circle who insists that she was out in a few days, with 'no bruising whatsoever'. Cosmetic surgery is like having a baby – you never remember all the gory details. (If we did, no sane woman would ever have a second child!) Some people bruise more than others. And if you bruised a lot from one procedure, it doesn't necessarily mean you'll be purple after the next thing you have done. The older you are, the more easily you bruise – blood vessels are made of collagen, which diminishes over time, and skin naturally thins with age.

WILL I NEED TO HAVE PHOTOGRAPHS TAKEN BEFORE SURGERY?

Preoperative photographs are usually mandatory. Many doctors take their own photos, using a digital camera. Typically, your surgeon will take a series of six to ten shots so that he can view the area of the face or body from various angles. Photos are used as a road map or blueprint for the surgery. These photographs will become part of your official medical chart, and they will be used to help plan your surgery. They will also become a valuable tool for both you and your doctor to compare your final result. It is easy to forget what your face, lips or hips looked like before an operation. Having these photos as documentation is a helpful reminder of the improvement (or lack of improvement) achieved.

Computer imaging is also a great tool. It is valuable as a visual aid to show you what you can expect. The ability to see an approximation of what your new profile might look like – with less nose and more chin, for instance – is compelling. It also teaches you to look at your face or upper and lower body as a cohesive, single unit, instead of singling out one feature you want to change. However, no doctor can guarantee the computer-generated results you see on a screen. These should be used only as a guideline. Surgery is not a perfect science – and it is not as simple as moving a mouse or cursor to take something away or shift it around.

NIP TIP
You can't always judge your doctor on how much bruising you get. It isn't the best predictor of how good the result will be. Some people become more black and blue than others; and some doctors have a heavier hand.

The Nuts and Bolts of Having Surgery

Cosmetic Beauty Calendar

January

Facelifts and big body-contouring procedures like tummy tucks are ideal for cold, dark, long January. You can stay in or cover up in cashmere scarves without feeling as if you're missing out. Everyone is overstuffed and overspent, and the social scene is quiet. You will have something to look forward to during the winter doldrums, besides the post-Christmas sales.

February

Plump up lips for Valentine's Day. The dead of winter is a great time to hide away after surgery. If you are short of a beau this year, pick a long weekend and have the lot done. February is a short month, so plan accordingly.

March

March is ideal to do the full lot – face, neck, eyes, brow! Filled with dreary weather and lacking in holidays and good cheer, March is a great time for rejuvenation and getting a jump-start on spring cleaning. Look out for Easter, though, which can come early.

April

Time to start thinking about summer holiday plans; the ski season has nearly passed, but golf is just beginning. If you want to bare a new body, lipo and breast implants are de rigueur. As hemlines rise and necklines plunge, evaluate your legs and décolleté. Thread veins, cellulite and unwanted hair may be on your agenda. Slough away dead skin for spring with peels and light devices.

May

Summer is just around the corner, but a little last-minute thigh contouring or neck redraping can work. It's getting late in the season for lasering or deeper peels. Races, graduations and garden parties will start cropping up. Don't wait until the first hint of pastels in Selfridges' windows to start planning.

June

It's wedding season, so mothers of the bride (and groom) should take notice. This month is a good time to have some work done if your children summer away, or if you are lucky enough to take off July and August. If your summer is booked up, you can still squeeze in a little tuck before you fly.

July

If you've waited all year to enjoy the seaside, pull out your sunhat, douse yourself with sunblock and put your beauty regime on hold. If your only holiday is summertime, plan to have your nose or chin done and look great for the first autumn leaves. Surgery is out for the in crowd. Hot and humid weather is a bad time in most places for anything that requires dressings and covering up. After surgery, sun exposure is forbidden anyway.

August

Early to mid-August is ideal for nipping for the back-to-school set. Teens line up to have their noses and breasts reduced during the summer. Schoolteachers and therapists pick August for the same reason. Business practically shuts down in Europe and America, as the whole world seems to be on holiday, including cosmetic surgeons. You can steal some privacy if the timing suits you, but plan ahead.

September

Eyelid surgery, Botox® and fillers are a good way to begin the season looking rested from your summer holiday. This is a busy month, crowded with back-to-school and work rituals, but the countryside is a lovely place to recover. Just after school starts is prime time for nips and tucks.

October

The ideal month for lifts of all kinds – of the face and the body. The transition from autumn to winter warrants a personal treat such as taking a decade off your face. There is still plenty of time to look great for the holidays if you move quickly.

November

It's getting late in the season for a facelift if you plan to entertain 20 relatives for Christmas dinner. Cool wintry winds keep you well preserved and cosy inside. Get your holiday shopping done before you go under the knife, or else you'll be too stressed to heal properly.

December

Emergency fillers, skin treatments and Botox® rule. Savvy women pop in for microdermabrasion or light treatments the day before a gala so that they glow. End-of-year cosmetic surgery is popular. Find a flexible doctor so that you can breeze in for a beauty shot when a party invitation arrives unexpectedly.

SURGERY BUDDIES

Going it alone can be an anxiety-ridden experience. Don't underestimate the importance of having a support system. The entire process can be traumatic. Tell at least one person you can trust and swear her to secrecy. Doing it with a girlfriend or sister is a good idea – but not always practical. Your schedules and budgets need to be simpatico to make it work. Women are intensely competitive with each other, so choose wisely. One of you will end up healing faster and looking better than the other, and that can put a damper on your relationship.

Fenella and Louisa get lifted
Friends since childhood, Fenella and Louisa plucked up the courage to have a little work done. Although they were both turning 6o, Fenella summered in Spain and loved to spend hours in her garden, which showed on her face, neck and hands. Louisa, on the other hand, never went in the sun and was quite unlined for her age. Going to a consultation together was a disaster waiting to happen. Fenella needed the works – a face- and necklift, browlift, upper and lower eyelids, and laser. Louisa could do with just a facelift and having some fat taken from her lower eyelids. They compared notes, and it got a little tense for a while. In the end, Fenella chickened out and Louisa went ahead and had surgery on her own. When she saw her friend's result, Fenella was inspired to reconsider. After some encouragement from yours truly, she did it too!

GETTING READY FOR THE BIG DAY

A satisfying cosmetic surgery experience is indeed possible with meticulous planning. The less you have to worry about during the days preceding your surgery, the more relaxed you can be. Make sure that kids and animals as well as lovers or partners are all taken care of. You'll be in no shape to take your Westie for a romp around the park or to do the school run for a while.

If your hair is very short, let it grow before face or neck surgery so that it is long enough to hide scars around the ears while they heal. You can have it cut when you are ready to face the world again. If you could do with losing a few pounds, to get the best result possible the time to do it is before surgery. Losing a stone after having a lift may cause the skin to loosen up more quickly than you anticipated, and then you will have blown your investment.

Make sure to tell your doctor about any medications you take, both prescription and over the counter. Your doctor may ask you to give up alcohol, caffeine, aspirin and aspirin-containing drugs, hormone replacements or birth control pills, and any medications that may cause blood clots and bruising. Do not take anything that can disrupt the clotting process, including vitamin E, aspirin and ibuprofen. You should not interrupt other medications you currently take – such as high blood pressure meds – unless your surgeon or anaesthetist instructs you to do so.

WHAT TO STOP BEFORE SURGERY

NOTE: Medications to be discontinued before and after surgery may include: tablets, capsules, elixirs, suppositories, injections, creams, gels, foams and cold medications. Always consult your doctor or pharmacist.

Anti-inflammatories (NSAIDs)
Aspirin, Nurofen, Advil, Anadin Ibuprofen, Arthrofen, Brufen, Brufen Retard, Cuprofen, Fenbid, Galprofen, Hedex Ibuprofen, Ibufem, Librofem, Mandafen, Manorfen, Migrafen, Motrin, Nurofen Plus, Obifen, Relcofen, Voltaren, Ibuprofen, Diclofenac, Naproxen, Angettes, Aspro, Caprin, Disprin, Nu-Seals Aspirin, Acoflam, Arthrotec, Defanac, Dicloflex, Diclomax, Diclovol, Diclozip, Econac, Fenactol, Flamatak, Flamrase, Flexotard, Lofensaid, Motifene, Rheumatac, Rhumalgan, Volsaid, Voltarol, Naprosyn

Cold medicines
Alka Seltzer, Alka-Seltzer XS

Anti-coagulants
Warfarin, Coumadin®, Jantoven®, Marevan®, Waran®

Plastic Makes Perfect

Your doctor may prescribe antibiotics and pain medication before surgery. Don't wait until you are sore and stiff to send your partner to get them, only to find that the chemist closed at six o'clock, so risking staying up all night throbbing. In some cases, your doctor will prescribe antibiotics to be taken prior to surgery, as a precaution, especially if you have a history of mitral valve prolapse (abnormality of the heart), a heart murmur or a hip or joint replacement. Tell your doctor if you have ever had an allergic reaction to any of the cephalosporins, penicillins or penicillin-like medicines. Keflex®/Cefalexin, Zithromax®, Ciproxin®/Ciprofloxacin, Floxapen®/Flucloxacillin or Augmentin may be given to guard against infections. They work by killing bacteria or preventing their growth. If you tend to get cold sores and are having facial surgery or a procedure around the mouth (such as lip enhancement or lasers), ask your doctor about taking an antiviral medication in

NIP TIP

If you are losing your hair or are worried about hair loss from face or browlift surgery, consider a course of Regaine® for Women 2% as a pre-emptive strike. It takes about four months to regrow hair, so factor that in to your plans. Ask your pharmacist for advice. See www.regaine.co.uk.

order to prevent eruptions. Zovirax® is available over the counter at chemists in a handy pump dispenser or a tube. Early treatment when you first feel a tingle can stop a cold sore dead in its tracks.

You will be instructed not to eat or drink after midnight before your surgery. You will be allowed to brush your teeth on the morning of surgery, without swallowing any water. If you tend to get sick from medications, or have a history of motion sickness, tell your anaesthetist ahead of time so that he or she can give you anti-nausea drugs during surgery. If you do get sick, it will be the thing you remember most about your recovery, and it can be easily avoided.

WHAT TO WEAR TO SURGERY

On the morning of your procedure, you can shower, but you must forego moisturiser, body lotion, make-up, hair gels and fragrance. You may be asked to remove nail varnish from fingers and/or toes. Forget contact lenses, but bring your glasses if you tend to bump into walls without them.

Wear only loose-fitting clothes that are easy to put on, button down the front and fit over bulky dressings. Pointy toes, lace-up boots and stilettos are out, since your feet and ankles will swell up like balloons after surgery. Trainers or a well-stretched-out pair of ballet flats are your best bet. Leave your valuables, such as watches, diamond studs, wedding bands, cash and Anya Hindmarch bags, at home. All jewellery must be removed anyway; fingers swell from the anaesthetic solution, which makes getting rings back on tricky. Hospitals are very unsafe

WHAT TO BRING

- Cosy nightgown that covers anything you would rather not expose
- Comfy tracksuit that zips down the front
- Sports bra with front fastening (if you can find one)
- Slippers or socks – hospitals are cold, damp places
- Small, soft toothbrush and toothpaste – so that you don't have to open too wide
- Oversized dark sunglasses with wide sides
- Large opaque scarf – challis or pashmina, not chiffon

places for personal items that can be easily pinched if left unattended. Basically, don't bring anything you can't afford to lose. (Even surgeons do this themselves.)

It is common to ooze, bleed, drip and leak after cosmetic surgery, so leave your favourite Hermès scarf or cashmere jumper at home. Think M&S, not couture. If you are going to be staying overnight in hospital, pack a small bag with only the bare essentials. For body procedures, if you were told to buy a support bra or compression garment (see page 149), bring these with you to hospital.

WHAT HAPPENS BEFORE SURGERY?

After checking into the hospital, and filling out an endless pile of forms, you will be ready to get going. It really helps to have someone with you, to curb your anxiety and to answer questions intelligently. Hospitals often don't run exactly on time, so you might bring some reading material to make the time pass more quickly if you have to hang around waiting to be called.

It is normal to be a nervous wreck before having surgery. In fact, if you don't feel a little scared, you probably haven't thought it through properly. The idea of going under the surgeon's knife is terrifying, especially if you have never done anything like this before. The anaesthetist will be your new best friend!

Once you are wheeled into the operating theatre, the anaesthetist will give you a small injection that will make you drowsy. This is likely to be the last thing you will remember, as within seconds you will be completely unconscious. The anaesthetic will be flowing to keep you comfortably asleep during the operation, while a device clipped on to your fingertip called a pulse oximeter will monitor your heart rate, blood pressure and breathing rate by the minute. When you wake, the procedure will be over and you will have virtually no sense of how much time has elapsed or any memory of the surgery (luckily).

NIP TIP
Stay away from magnifying mirrors. In fact, avoid looking at yourself in the mirror as much as possible. It's like dieting: if you jump on a scale every single day, you won't see the pounds roll off.

The Nuts and Bolts of Having Surgery

After surgery, you will be taken to a recovery room, where you will be closely monitored by nurses (you hope). You may be given extra oxygen, and your breathing and heart functions will be observed closely. In most cases, you will be wheeled or, if you are able, walk (slowly and with some assistance) out of the hospital or clinic to a waiting car. Make arrangements to have someone take you home after surgery and stay with you for the first 24 hours.

Once you get home, go directly to bed. Change into comfortable clothes or a robe and settle down to rest. Create a comforting, soothing environment to promote healing. Relaxing aromatherapy or candles (lavender, rosemary, eucalyptus, orange, lemon) can set a calming mood. Set yourself up in the room where you will be staying for most of the next few days, preferably on the same level as a toilet and sink to avoid dealing with stairs. Skid-free socks or slippers are good if you have wooden floors.

This is not the time to snuggle into your Frette bed linen. You may ooze, leak or drain on to your duvet, sheets and pillows. To avoid soiling, use waterproof pillow protectors. Disposable puppy-training pads, also called chux, are great on a bed if you have had any bodywork done. These are typically blue or green plastic on one side and thick absorbent white cotton on the other.

Rest inside for at least the first 48 hours. You will feel drowsy from the anaesthetics and may have muscle aches, a sore throat from where the airway tube was placed if you had a general anaesthetic, dizziness or headaches. If you are unlucky, you may also have nausea and vomiting, so keep a basin nearby just in case.

You will have been given local injections into the areas around your incisions during the procedure and as they wear off over the first 24 hours, you may need prescription pain medication. The painkillers used post-op include Celecoxib and morphine for serious pain, and Co-Proxamol and codeine for moderate pain. After the first few days, you can switch to over-the-counter pain medication, or nothing at all. There are three main analgesics that you can buy over the counter: paraceta-

Plastic Makes Perfect

mol (acetomeniphen), ibuprofen and aspirin. These are available either on their own or combined with codeine (or a similar codeine-like product). Unlike ibuprofen and aspirin, paracetamol does not have the possible side-effect of bleeding. Although these are available without a prescription, your doctor or pharmacist can instruct you on the proper dose for you.

To reduce swelling and discomfort, apply cold compresses consistently, keeping your head and torso elevated. Compresses can take the form of a bowl of ice and a flannel or gauze pads that are dipped into cool water.

Finding a comfortable position in bed or a chair and learning to sleep on your back presents new challenges. Call in reinforcements in the form of extra pillows and rolled-up blankets to bolster your neck or elevate your knees, as needed.

You may be light-headed after anaesthesia, so avoid rising from a sitting position or getting out of bed too quickly. If you have had a tummy tuck or a bodylift, using a cane or the back of a chair to help you get up out of bed can be a godsend. Keep one hand on something stationary and the other hand free to steady yourself in case you feel dizzy, as if you are on a sloop off the coast of the Bahamas.

For the first 48 hours, the risk of haematoma (blood clot) is greatest. After ten days, the risk drops considerably. Find out how to manage any unforeseen symptoms that may arise, such as excessive bleeding or leaking. Make sure you know what to expect after surgery so that there are no surprises.

Your doctor's staff should review with you the specifics of what you can and cannot do before and after surgery in terms of medications, foods, bathing, exercise, sex, etc. These are

OVER-THE-COUNTER POST-SURGERY PAINKILLERS

- Panadol
- Tylenol
- Paracetamol
- Paramol
- Paracodol
- Anadin paracetamol
- Solpadeine

NIP TIP
After torso surgeries (tummy tucks, bodylifts, thighlifts) a portable lifting cushion can be a lifesaver – like an ejector seat to help you lift your sore, bloated body out of a chair. See www.otstores.co.uk.

The Nuts and Bolts of Having Surgery

75

non-negotiable. Generally, aerobics, jogging, weight training and sports are discouraged for at least three weeks after any surgical procedure. Any activity that elevates your heart rate can increase swelling and cause bleeding and pressure on your suture lines. Also find out about driving (meaning you at the wheel) and flying in an aeroplane. The risk of getting a train that stalls because of 'leaves on the track' may also be too great. You may need to plan to have someone drive you to your doctor to have your stitches removed.

Major swelling will go down within the first few weeks, but you may be swollen for several months or longer. Gravity tends to cause fluids to settle at the lowest point on the body. For example, the tip of the nose takes the longest to settle after a nasal operation; ankles bear the brunt of the swelling from lower leg liposuction. As swelling goes down, you will start to feel your nerve endings coming back to life. You will feel some tingling, like tiny fingers waking up the area that has been traumatised.

THE FIRST 24 HOURS

- Do not drink. Although you may be dying for a few glasses of Chablis, it will make you swell.
- Do not smoke (anything), and ban all smokers from lighting up around you. Secondhand smoke or 'passive smoke' can interfere with healing.
- Avoid placing a phone to your ear if you have had facial surgery – germs cause infection.
- Keep a sports bottle next to your bed. Drink fluids: water, juices, low-sodium broth, decaffeinated tea, fruit smoothies.
- If necessary, sip liquids through a straw or use a toddler's sippy cup (don't laugh – it works).
- Eat a soft, bland diet and work your way up to solid foods.
- Avoid salty, spicy, greasy foods, and preservatives – curry and chilli are off limits.
- Use a bed tray to serve meals.
- Premoistened baby wipes are great for freshening up until you can bathe.
- Organise your medications in a pillbox by your bedside, clearly labelled to avoid mistaking one for another.

Plastic Makes Perfect

You should be able to pass water readily, and check that your bowels are functioning normally. Constipation is common after having an anaesthetic and when taking some pain medications such as codeine. Your doctor may recommend a stool softener like DulcoEase™ or some prune juice to keep things moving along without straining. Straining can cause tension on stitches, and incisions may bleed or loosen up.

Infections from the surgery itself are actually quite rare. As well as a course of antibiotics given before and/or after surgery, you may be given a dose of antibiotics by injection or intravenously during surgery. This class of antibiotics may be taken on a full or empty stomach, but if they upset your stomach, it may help to take them with food.

Be on the lookout for signs of infection near incisions: increased swelling, redness, high fever, warmth, bleeding or other discharge. The older you are, the longer wounds take to heal. Any unusual or severe symptoms – heavy uncontrollable bleeding, a high fever, intense throbbing, sudden pain followed by significant swelling – should be reported to your doctor or his nurse straight away. If you don't get a response in a timely fashion, and are very worried, call your GP or go to the nearest NHS hospital.

If you have had a facelift, breast surgery or tummy tuck, clear plastic drainage tubes may be used to prevent fluid from collecting. You will be shown how to empty your drains and record the amount of blood or fluid that fills up the little bulb each time so that your doctor can decide how long to keep them in. Typically, drains are removed within a few days or a week. You will want them out as quickly as possible, but they are removed in a way that can make your heart skip a beat or two.

NIP TIP
A hose that attaches to the tap or showerhead can come in handy for washing your hair in the sink or bath. These are commonly available in baby or nursery departments, and in pet shops (for bathing small dogs indoors). If you have had a facial procedure, dilute your shampoo or use baby shampoo, and use a spray-on detangler to make hair easier to comb through. Use only a wide toothcomb or fingers – do not brush or comb through hair.

WASH CYCLE

Your suture lines should be kept clean and dressings dry and intact. For example, if you have a plaster splint on your nose, you cannot take a shower because you will get the splint wet, which would cause it to loosen or fall off. In most cases, you will be able to have a bath or shower in the first one to three days. You may need some assistance with bathing and washing your hair. A shower or bathing cap will keep scalp sutures dry. Your first shower may leave you feeling as if your sutures are going to pop open, but your body heals faster than you think. After large procedures, a safety chair, bench or handrail in the shower or bath is also helpful.

Avoid using water that is too hot or too cold; lukewarm or tepid is best. Any treated body parts will be numb, so you can easily and unwittingly burn yourself if you don't test the water properly. The scalp can be especially vulnerable; avoid using a hairdryer or any other hair appliance close to your head, and keep it on a low setting.

HOME SWEET HOME

Your recovery will take place in the comfort of your own home, causing less disruption to your lifestyle and schedule than the time spent in hospital. For the most part, husbands and partners – and men in general – make really bad caretakers. If possible, send them out of town, or golfing or fishing with their mates. Mothers, sisters and daughters are usually better. Women are programmed to be caretakers. You need a little TLC and a good supply of CDs, DVDs, glossy magazines and books to get you through the early days of soreness.

RECOVERY MASTER PLAN

The more extensive your surgery, the longer you will have to wait to resume normal activities. Here are approximate timings you might expect:

- Home sweet home: same day or next day
- Shower or bathe: 1–3 days
- Washing your hair: 1–2 days
- Dressing removal: 1–5 days
- Suture removal: 3–10 days
- Staple removal: 5–10 days
- Draining tube removal: 1–5 days
- Bruising: up to 3 weeks
- Make-up: 7–10 days
- Hair colour: 3–6 weeks
- Exercise: 2–3 weeks
- Flying: 4–10 days
- Sex: 3 weeks or when you're ready

Plastic Makes Perfect

Before you see the changes you are expecting, you may look strange to yourself. Typically you will look your worst for the first three days. This is quite normal and not a cause for alarm. It is not easy to look at the immediate effects of surgery, especially when your natural expectation is that you have done something to improve your appearance. As the first few weeks progress, your new look will emerge. After two or three months, you will look great. After four to six months, you will look fabulous.

Rose's mother's face

A few days after her facelift, Rose got quite a scare. When she looked in the mirror she was a bit dizzy from the pain pill and thought she saw her mother staring back at her. Rose was horrified for about ten seconds, until she realised that her mother, even when she was younger, had always had a plump face with chipmunk cheeks and tiny slits for eyes. And because of all the swelling that's exactly what Rose looked like.

THE COLOUR PURPLE

The good news is that with new techniques and medications, there is less trauma after cosmetic surgery than there used to be. Bruising can last for up to three weeks after any invasive procedure. If you have fair or thin skin, it may take longer to subside. Some procedures yield little bruising but a lot of swelling. Everyone's response is different. Tell your doctor about any history of excessive bleeding, heavy menstrual periods or if you are taking blood thinners. Smokers tend to bruise more. Delicate skin (such as the eyelid area) bruises more easily, and the side or area that requires the most work may also bruise more. This accounts for why you may end up with more discolouration and swelling on one breast over the other, or on one cheek, eye and so on. Older skin tends to bruise more too, although scars are usually not as thick. Less fat padding coupled with years of sun exposure weakens collagen and blood vessels, so any trauma can cause leakage of blood from the vein into the skin to form a bruise.

The Nuts and Bolts of Having Surgery

Bruising tends to get worse before it gets better. You may see bruising straight away, or you may wake up the morning after and be shocked. You will look your worst after about three days, when swelling comes to a peak, and then everything will speed up. After that, your body will start to break down the bruising. The course of bruising varies from one person to another, but for most people, it takes about three weeks to go from blue or purple, to spotty green and yellow. (For tips on camouflage make-up, see page 286.)

RECOVERY REMEDIES

To make your recovery process more comfortable, I recommend the following handy, helpful and often essential items. Every little bit helps – even something as small as having the right pillow or a clever way to put cold compresses on your swelling can make a real difference. We have come a long way from bog-standard bags of frozen peas! (Although in a crisis, they still work too.)

Note Do not use anything on an open wound, unless instructed to do so by your doctor, and do not attempt to use any of the devices and products below without your doctor's permission.

How you scar is determined by your genetic package, like the colour of your skin and the texture of your hair. It usually has nothing to do with your surgeon's skill or the technique used. Paying attention to skin pigmentation is important, and a preoperative skin assessment could yield significant findings.

Healing devices

Ivivi Technologies A revolutionary device that utilises micro-electrical currents to increase blood flow, which speeds healing. There are varieties for breast procedures, a facial unit, and another for post-tummy tuck or bodylift, to cut down on pain and tenderness. Highly recommended for level 3–4 on the Ouch Factor Scale (see page 91), and especially for bigger surgeries; see www.ivivitechnologies.com.

Natragel® Must-have hydrogel patches to calm and hydrate compromised skin. They come as a full face mask or circles for eyelids or around the mouth, and can be customised to fit any area. Found in high-end spas and clinics; see www.natragel.com.

Reusable hot/cold pack May be used for both cold and hot therapy to reduce swelling, bruising and stinging from peels, Botox®, fillers, face and eyelid surgery. Keep a few in the fridge so they are cold when you need to switch off (at pharmacies nationwide).

Comfort and convenience

Thermometer To take your temperature to check if you have a fever, which could be a sign of infection. At chemists.

Female urinal or bed pan To use after body procedures when it is hard to get up out of bed. At chemists.

Memory foam wedge pillow Comfortable squishy pillows can cushion your head in bed, help you avoid muscle tension and body aches, and keep body parts elevated that need to be (knees, ankles, head, etc.). See www.putnams.co.uk.

NIP TIP
To avoid dark or grey roots showing up after a face or browlift, ColorMark® is a brilliant temporary liquid touch-up. It is real hair colour in 12 shades that you apply where your roots are noticeable – around the hairline and your parting – until you can have your whole head coloured again. See www.color-markpro.com.

Wound care

Biafine® WDE An opaque white healing cream ointment used for post-op wounds. See www.biafine.com.

Polyfax ointment Polymyxin B, a clear gel in a tube that is a lifesaver for keeping wounds and scars soft and supple. Also called Polysporin, Bacitracin®, Neosporin®. Found in pharmacies.

Auriderm XO® Gel Nannosome vitamin K plus C and E formula, applied twice a day to speed up bruising. Also comes in a stick for easy application. See www.auriga-int.com.

Bactroban and Flamazine Topical antibiotic creams used to heal and prevent infection, especially for smokers, whose oxygen supply to the skin is cut off. Ask your pharmacist.

Nelson's arnica cream and Arnica 30c tablets Soothing and healing arnica cream in a tube or tiny pellets you pop under your tongue to

The Nuts and Bolts of Having Surgery

help reduce bruising and swelling. See www.hollandandbarrett.com.

Sinecch® Industrial-strength arnica capsules. Can be used after injections as well as after surgery, so keep some in stock. See www.sinecch.com.

Vitamedica Healing Supplements Program Nutritional support used by American cosmetic surgeons to minimise inflammation and bruising, with Bromelain and arnica. See www.vitamedica.com.

Luxe healers

When a £5 tube of Polyfax just won't do it for you, and you need a little glamour to get you through recovery, try these lovely, soothing healers.

La Prairie Cellular Nurturing Complex A luxurious duo of healing therapies for sensitive, traumatised skin. See www.laprairie.com.

Crème de La Mer Concentrate Designed for fragile, post-trauma skin to complement the skin's own natural healing process. See www.cremedelamer.com.

Elizabeth Arden Eight Hour Cream Classic healing balm, now in a body formula too for superdry, itchy post-liposuction legs, hips and tummies. See www.elizabetharden.com.

Clinique Cx Rapid Recovery Cream Soothes sensitive skin and calms inflammation. See www.clinique.co.uk.

Akademikliniken Pure Recovery Crème Vitamin-loaded formula for post-op, laser and peels, with antioxidant protection. See www.akademiklinikenshop.se.

Jurlique Herbal Recovery Gel Highly concentrated antioxidant mixture without chemicals or preservatives. See www.jurlique.com.

Jo Malone Vitamin E Gel Sumptuous multi-tasking vitamin E concentrated gel. See www.jomalone.com.

> ### MASSAGE – THE COSMETIC SURGEON'S SECRET WEAPON
>
> Have you ever noticed that when you don't like a scar or your skin feels too taut, most cosmetic surgeons tell you to massage gently? Sometimes it is just because they're not sure what else to say because it's just going to take some time to heal and they know you are anxious. Generally, massaging gives you something to do, and some feel that it does speed up healing by improving the circulation. You feel better because you are being proactive about your aftercare.

THE HEALING PHASE

It is normal to feel tired, anxious or depressed in the days or weeks following your operation. Stress causes hormones to be released that can cause headaches, high blood pressure, sleeplessness and irritability. Your hormone levels change after surgery and you may start to feel sad or scared that you will never look like yourself again. These feelings should pass eventually.

The aftermath of a procedure can bring on feelings of depression and let-down. The period immediately after surgery is a particularly vulnerable time for many women. You will not look or feel like yourself, but this is only a temporary condition. There is a phenomenon called the 'third-day blues' – which means that on the third day after surgery, you have regained your stamina and are feeling better, but you still don't look so good. Many people don't really understand how banged up and bruised they may be after surgery. The reality is that recovering from surgery will shut down your life for a few weeks. The physical trauma to the body is also coupled with the emotional impact.

NIP AND TALK

Despite the huge increase in the use of cosmetic enhancements, in many circles no one really wants to admit to it. To tell or not to tell – that is the question. Most British women still keep at least some of their adventures under the knife a secret from even their closest friends. In the UK, it is common not to tell husbands, children or parents. Some of my clients don't even tell their long-time partners, although I think in this day and age that is a stretch.

With bodywork, you can easily keep it a total secret. Just say you've lost some weight or hired a personal trainer. But above the neck, the issue gets fiddly. It is naïve to expect that after having a facelift with eyelid work and a browlift, no one will know you have had anything done. Changing your hairstyle can create a diversion, but in the era of makeover television, someone would had to have been living on a remote desert island to be completely in the dark about what it is likely you have had done. If the op has made you look different, such as a nasal surgery, a chin implant or a full facelift with the works, people who know you well and see you on a regular basis will suspect that you have had something done. The days when you could explain your sudden good fortune of looking fab by telling your admirers you've just had a nice holiday or spa retreat are long gone. In New York, you have to watch out for nosy doormen. It is nearly impossible to sneak past them in bandages and black eyes, and they tend to have loose lips. In England, it's the gardeners who will tell all your secrets as they work elsewhere in your village. Hairstylists and make-up artists, although sympathetic to your cause, often have an uncanny knack for relinquishing precious personal details that you might not have expected them to divulge. If you find out that someone you have sworn to secrecy has spilled the beans, you have a right to be royally peeved.

My philosophy is simple: tell a little, keep a little. You can deny everything, but some people will figure it out eventually. Lying outright if you obviously look different can make you the unwitting topic of conversation around the water cooler. If you work in the city around mostly men, you might get away with it – men are much less observant than women. But if you spend your time in the company of women, or work in an environment saturated with females (or gay males), you'll be out of luck. Do what celebs do – downsize. I advise my clients to involve as few people as possible in the whole process and not to reveal everything they have done. Unless you are really keen to tell all, keep at least some of the details to yourself. You can say you've had a little laser when you've really done the works. For example, a full facelift sounds less major if you call it a 'mini tuck'; or you could say you've had your eyebags removed when in fact you have had your eyelids, brows and neck lifted all in one go.

Another good explanation: tell them you have taken a lover! That will really give your female friends something to be jealous about.

Plastic Makes Perfect

The ultimate compliment after any type of cosmetic surgery or treatment is to be told you look well rested. This shows that people notice that you look good, and at the same time that you are not sporting a sign that tells the world you've had some surgical help.

The mumps and the mother-in-law
A few years ago, Sarah's husband visited his mother and when he came home, said that she was quite swollen from having mumps. Sarah thought this sounded rather odd, since mumps were really a childhood illness and not likely in a woman of nearly 70. When Sarah went to see her mother-in-law, it was clear that it was not the mumps at all; rather, she had had a facelift and hadn't told anyone about it. She might have fooled her son, but Sarah knew better. Perhaps her mother-in-law thought she could get away with such a lame excuse, but people are much more switched on today. Sarah thought, 'Anything I come up with has to be more believable than the mumps.'

THE LADY DOTH PROTEST TOO MUCH

I don't blame anyone for wanting to keep her cosmetic enhancements a private matter. Every woman is entitled to a little mystery, but come on! I often hear some of my clients doing interviews that make me giggle. Most celebs who state unequivocally 'I would never have poison injected in my face' and go pale at even the mere suggestion that they would ever consider 'going under the knife' are not always being entirely honest.

Think about it this way: if you're on the wrong side of 50, something has started to sag and wrinkle. I guarantee it. It's a scientific fact of life, a truism that needs no other proof than to ask any woman in the free world. Celebrity diehards who condemn their counterparts for their forays into silicone and surgery may end up singing a different tune when they are asked to play the ageing mother or wretched mother-in-law to an actress who is only a dozen or so years younger. How many times have we read the headlines about some starlet who says she

The Nuts and Bolts of Having Surgery

might consider cosmetic surgery in the future! Usually this is an indication or one of two things: either she has had some (or quite a lot) already and is trying to redeem herself from having condemned it in the past, or she is doesn't want to condemn it entirely when she may have to rely on it in the future, therefore essentially preparing the media and her public for the inevitability of her after look. Then there are celebs who admit to having a bit of Botox® or breast implants (as if we couldn't tell), and then retract it quickly after the news is plastered all over the BBC and gets picked up in media outlets all over the world.

FIVE GREATEST CELEBRITY LIES

- 'It's in my genes.'
- 'I would consider it in the future.'
- 'All I've had done is a bit of Botox®.'
- 'I take loads of vitamins and herbs.'
- 'I'm just lucky, I guess.'

Ask The Beauty Junkie®

How do I know who will administer the anaesthetic during my surgery?

In most cases, you will not be able to choose your own anaesthetist, even though the skill of the anaesthetist may be just as important as the surgeon's. Most surgeons work with one or several anaesthetists at each hospital where they operate. Which anaesthetist will be assigned to your individual case will depend on the day of your operation.

When should I get a second opinion if I am not happy after my surgery?

You need to give yourself time to heal and to allow for things to settle. Invariably, what you see at three weeks will have gone away on its own by three months; or you may start to like it. It is normal to feel anxious if you are not healing quickly and to jump to the conclusion that there is a problem. Keep a list of what you don't like, and as time goes on, cross off each item that resolves itself. If there are some remaining issues that your doctor has not fully explained, you can always get a second opinion later.

Can I get compensation if I don't get a good result from cosmetic surgery?

According to the insurance industry, over £1 million is paid out on negligence claims for cosmetic surgery that has gone wrong each year. However, being unhappy with the results of your surgery is not a reason to go to court. Compensation will be awarded only if there has been serious medical negligence that causes long-term or permanent injury or trauma that is well documented. A possible consequence of surgery such as too much fat taken out of one thigh or a droopy eyelid is not actionable. In addition, the process of filing a lawsuit against a physician is not a pleasant one, and it will take years and a considerable amount of your time and possibly legal fees to see your claim through.

Is it safe to have surgery and go home the same day?

The worldwide trend in cosmetic surgery is towards ambulatory surgery centres where you can have your procedure done and go home after a few hours. Faster-acting anaesthetics and simpler techniques have made this possible, and people appreciate the option of having surgery outside a proper hospital setting where they have to stay overnight. Outside the UK, many countries have outpatient surgery facilities, and physicians often operate their own clinics as well. The big advantage is that privately run centres are often more patient-friendly than traditional hospitals, and offer better service and more attentive after care. Unfortunately, this is not commonly done in the UK at the present time.

If you have one thing done, do you have to keep on doing more things?

Think of it this way. If you have highlights done to make your hair blonde, there is no Public Bill before Parliament that states that you have to keep lightening your hair. However, the new hair that grows will not be blonde. Injectables and laser treatments work in a similar way. If you have one Botox® treatment and don't go back in four months when your muscle activity returns to normal, the wrinkles will return. However, this does not apply to surgical procedures. If you have a facelift, the effects should last for years. If you never have another facelift done, you will always look younger and tighter because you had the first one. Facial surgery does not accelerate the ageing process.

Part II
MAKING THE CUT: LIFTS AND LIPO

Cosmetic surgery has two separate and not necessarily mutually exclusive missions. On one hand, it can beautify a feature (for instance, by reducing the size of your nose or enhancing your cheekbones). On the other hand, it can restore something to an earlier state, as in anti-ageing procedures (lifting droopy brows or tucking a saggy chin). The former tends to be done in your younger years; the latter is to be considered when you start seeing changes you do not appreciate.

Ageing is a bummer: you gain fat cells where you probably don't need any more, and you lose fat where it actually served a purpose, such as plumping up the hollows around your eyes and holding up your cheeks. Breasts get fattier as we age, but the rest of the body goes pear-shaped, which sounds as if it might even things out but it doesn't really. More fatty tissue in your breasts makes them heavier, and stretches out thinning skin, so breasts become bigger and droopier, just like your bottom.

Both your soft tissue and your facial bones change over the years. Cosmetic surgeons pay close attention to both. Generally, the first step may include procedures that build volume where bone has been lost, such as fillers. The second step involves procedures that lift, reposition and reduce the skin, fat and musculature that have lost elasticity.

In theory, surgeons need to make a scar for two basic reasons:

- to excise or take out skin
- to gain access to deeper tissues.

To determine if surgery is the best solution for you, think about whether you have extra bits of skin to remove (such as hanging upper eyelids, a loose neck or a floppy belly). The next test is whether any deeper tissues (such as muscles, fascia that covers the muscles, cartilage, bone, etc.) need to be tightened, elevated, moved around or reduced to accomplish your goals.

OUCH FACTOR

Everyone has a different pain tolerance, which is often dictated in part by your cultural background. The amount of discomfort you experience will depend on many other factors as well, including how deep the procedure goes, the tissues involved and how much anaesthetic you are given. Most cosmetic surgeries are actually very tolerable, but it's not a walk in the park. Some amount of discomfort is to be expected. The more extensive the surgery, the worse you will feel. In the descriptions of different cosmetic surgeries in the following chapters, I have indicated the level of pain you can expect according to my Ouch Factor Scale.

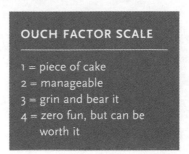

OUCH FACTOR SCALE

1 = piece of cake
2 = manageable
3 = grin and bear it
4 = zero fun, but can be
    worth it

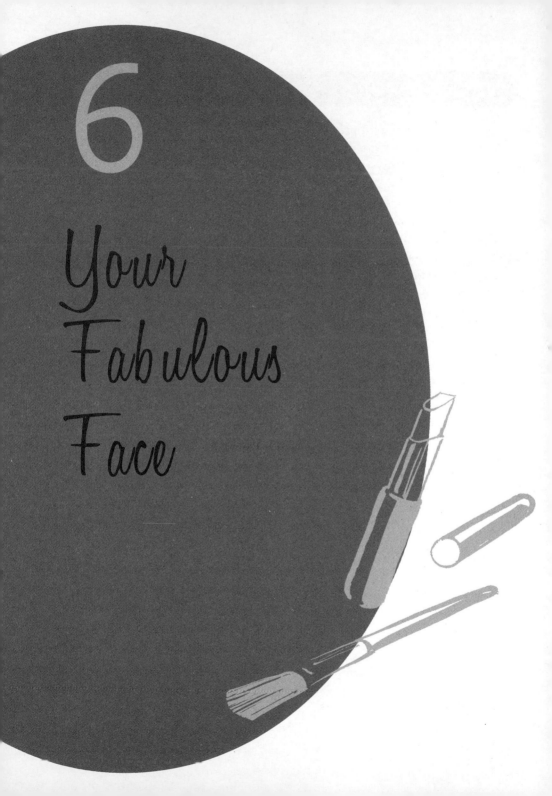

6

Your Fabulous Face

W hat can be done when a tight ponytail just doesn't do it any more and your chins seem to have a mind of their own? Nothing else takes the years off like a lift. No miracle cream or beam in a box, and nothing that comes in a syringe either. These treatments all help forestall the need for lifting, and preserve the results après the lift, but they are just not up to snuff when it comes to serious skin sagging.

EYELID LIFT

If you can only have one anti-ageing surgery, the best 'bang for the buck' is eyelid surgery. It offers the most in terms of rejuvenating your whole face and making you look youthful, refreshed and radiant. It changes your expression (in a good way), gives you a doe-like, open-eyed and engaging appearance, and delivers with a minimum of fuss, pain, visible scars and downtime.

Droopy or puffy lower eyelids often run in families, and are as common in men as they are in women; ditto for upper eyelids that tend to hang over your lashes. So if your father has to squint to see you, it may be a sign of things to come.

What it does

When the fat pad that cushions the eye begins to pull away from the bone of the lower eye and sag, it creates puffiness commonly referred to as bags. Sagging upper eyelids cause hooding, where the skin becomes heavier and fuller. It may seem as if your eyelids are at half-mast when you are wide awake. Eyelid surgery can reduce droopy or hooded eyelids, restore the contours and eliminate protruding fat bags under the eyes. It won't do much for wrinkles and crow's feet – it's all about skin removal, fat removal or repositioning and muscle tightening.

Your Fabulous Face

Concern Wrinkles and furrows.
Solution Zap tiny crow's feet and deep lines with muscle-relaxing injections and resurfacing (think lasers and chemical peels).

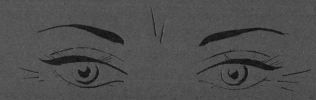

Concern Drooping or hooded eyelids.
Solution Botox® into your squinting muscles (in your crow's feet area) can lift heavy eyelids and give you a more wide-eyed look.

Concern Hollows under the eyes from fat loss.
Solution Thinner fillers which can plump up the valleys and crevices.

Concern Under-eye dark circles.
Solution Filler injections, which thicken the skin so that the bluish colour is less obvious and you look less tired.

Concern Under-eye bags from fatty deposits.
Solution The fat can be repositioned or removed. This is a surgical procedure.

Concern Over-plucked brows.
Solution Eyebrow transplants using your own hairs (from your head), but they grow as if the follicles are still on your scalp, so they require frequent pruning.

Concern Sparse eyelashes.
Solution Temporary eyelash extensions can be dramatic and seductive – high maintenance but worth it for a special look.

The procedure

The procedure may be performed under twilight or general anaesthetic, and you can do it as a day case to avoid spending the night in hospital. The most common technique for the lower eyelid area involves making an incision adjacent to the lower lashes. The skin and muscle are lifted to remove a small amount of fat. Excess skin and muscle are trimmed from the lower lid. If you just have fatty deposits, the fat can be removed from the inside of the eye without a visible scar. Upper eyelid surgery involves making an elliptical incision across the eyelid crease, in the natural skin fold, to follow the shape of your eyelids. The excess skin of the upper eyelid and fatty tissue are removed, along with a thin strip of muscle to give the eyelid crease more definition. Presto – you can apply eye shadow again!

Time in operating theatre

One to three hours.

Post-op effects and recovery time

Some swelling and bruising is to be expected for about a week. Keeping your head elevated with extra pillows helps encourage swelling to travel downwards. Cold compresses for the first 48 hours help. As the anaesthetic wears off, you may feel a slight burning sensation. Fine sutures are typically removed after three to five days. For seven to ten days, the area will need to be cleaned and the eyes may feel sticky, itchy and sore. You may need to use drops or a lubricant, especially at night-time. Contact lenses cannot be worn for one to two weeks. Avoid alcohol, which dries out the eyes and causes fluid retention. You should wear sunglasses because the eye area will be sensitive to sun, wind and other irritants for several weeks.

Risks

Lack of sufficient tears, thyroid problems, hypertension, cardiovascular disease and diabetes may increase your risks. If you have dry eyes before surgery, the problem may be the same or worse afterwards. Minor complications may include temporary double or blurred vision for a few days, a gritty sensation in the eye, excessive tearing and a slight asymmetry. Severe complications may include difficulty in closing your eyes completely, raised scars and an ectropion, where the lower lid is pulled down. A more serious but rare complication is bleeding behind the eye.

How long it lasts

Surgery may need to be repeated in about ten years. If it is just fatty deposits that are removed, excess skin may need to be removed at a later stage.

Minimum spend

£2,500–5,000.

Optimum age

Depending on your genes, 35 and up (eyebags often run in families).

Ouch factor

2.

What is the alternative?

Injections (Botox® and its cousins) and lasers such as plasma skin regeneration and fractional resurfacing can improve lines and crow's feet. Fillers such as Restylane®, HydraFill® and fat can camouflage deepened tear troughs. Thermage® can be used around the eyelids to shrink excess skin.

What it does

A browlift tightens loose skin, or may remove excess skin to smooth out forehead wrinkling. The eyebrows are yanked up into a slightly higher position, creating a more pleasing arch and opening up a crowded eyelid area. The muscles that cause deep vertical frown lines to form between the brows may also be removed, which can take you from looking cross all the time to appearing relaxed and content. A browlift is usually combined with upper and/or lower eyelid surgery or a facelift.

The procedure

There are many variations, but it is the endoscopic browlift that is most commonly done today. The endoscopic forehead lift uses three tiny incisions within the scalp. An endoscope – a small wand with a camera on the end connected to a monitor – is inserted so that the surgeon has a clear view of the muscles and tissues beneath the skin. The forehead is lifted and the muscles and underlying tissues are removed or released. The eyebrows may also be lifted and secured into their higher position beneath the surface of the skin. For a coronal browlift the incision is made slightly behind the natural hairline, running from ear to ear across your head, where a hair band or headset sits. If your hairline is high, the incision may be placed just at the hairline, to lower your hairline.

Time in operating theatre

One to three hours.

Post-op effects and recovery time

Stitches or staples are removed within a week. You will be able to shower and shampoo your hair within a couple of days. There may be numbness and temporary pulling around the incision. If you are prone to headaches, you may be treated with a longer-acting local anaesthestic during surgery as a preventive measure. Swelling and bruising may also affect the cheeks and eyes. As the nerves heal, the scalp may begin to itch, and may continue to do so for up to six months.

Risks

The nerves that control brow movement may be injured on one or both sides, which may result in an inability to raise the eyebrows or wrinkle the forehead, and numbness. This is usually a temporary condition, but may be permanent in rare cases. A widened scar may result, which may have to be revised. Some of the hair around the incisions may thin out, but normal growth usually resumes within a few months.

How long it lasts

Semi-permanent, five to ten years.

Minimum spend

£2,500–5,000.

Optimum age

Browlifts are typically done in the forties and up. If you have a low brow genetically, you may be a candidate earlier.

Ouch factor

2.

What is the alternative?

Botox®, Botox®, Botox® – the number of browlifts being done has been greatly reduced by the advent of Botox®. Generally, the time to do a browlift is when Botox® stops performing for you.

Temple worship

Called a lateral browlift or temple lift, a more diagonally directed lift can produce a swept-away look from the outer arch of the eyebrow to the temples. It can also lift your cheek skin and fat to restore a chiselled look. The procedure may be performed through a vertical incision behind your hairline or with small slits using an endoscope to lift the tissues under the skin. Tread lightly in this area – one too many temporal lifts may cause you to look a bit like a cat.

NIP TIP

Look in the mirror and take a pencil and hold it over one eyebrow; then extend it to the other eyebrow. Which one is higher? Most women over 40 have some form of asymmetry of their brows. This can be reduced with clever Botox® to lower or raise one brow to even them, or a browlift to raise the lower side.

Endotine® fixation

An Endotine® is an ingenious little absorbable implant used to fix areas of the forehead, brow and mid-face in place during a surgical lift. The original model is a triangular-shaped piece that keeps your brows where your surgeon puts them during a browlift. Over six months or so, it dissolves. Other variations have tiny tines that allow the surgeon to clamp on to a wide area with the holding power to tack up your cheek skin to give you cheekbones and smooth out nose-to-mouth creases. With this device, a cheeklift is usually done through an incision in the lower eyelid. Once the implant is absorbed, the tissue is wedged in place, presumably because of scar tissue forming. The downside is that you can feel the ridge of the implant in your scalp until it dissolves. See www.coaptsystems.com.

Your Fabulous Face

CHIN AUGMENTATION

What it does

Mentoplasty (also called genioplasty) involves the augmentation or reshaping of the chin. It is performed by inserting an implant under the skin. The implant builds up the chin and jawline to give the face a more balanced appearance. To add to a facial contour, the material is implanted deep below the skin and secured with permanent stitches into surrounding tissues, so that it cannot move around. There are many implant materials, shapes and sizes available, including silicone and elastomer. Facial implants are made from solid and semi-solid materials, unlike gel- or saline-filled breast implants.

The procedure

Most often, the incision is made under the chin in the crease and closed with sutures that are removed in five days. If the incision is inside the mouth, it is closed with absorbable sutures that later dissolve, but this is less common as there is a greater risk of infection. Your chin may be taped to minimise swelling, and you will wear a very unglamorous stretchy elastic around your head.

Time in operating theatre

One to two hours.

Post-op effects and recovery time

The area may feel tight and stiff, and moving your mouth can be a challenge. Apply cold compresses. Difficulty in talking, eating and smiling for several days is normal. You may be on a liquid diet until the stitches inside your mouth heal. Sutures under the chin are taken out after five to seven days. For several weeks avoid contact sports or any activity that may result in the face being jarred or bumped, such as travelling on the tube at rush hour or attending a football match.

Risks

Possible complications include the implant working its way up to the skin's surface, tightening of the scar tissue that distorts the implant, asymmetry and bone erosion. The implant can shift out of alignment or be placed improperly, in which case you may need a second operation to put it right. If you get an infection, the implant may have to be removed and replaced at a later date. Long-term numbness is a potential complication. In rare cases, pain, nerve weakness and nerve damage can occur if the implant is resting on one of your facial nerves. If your mouth looks off centre or slightly crooked, or you find yourself drooling, march back to your surgeon and find out why. This can be a sign that something has gone awry.

How long it lasts

Results are permanent; however, an implant may shift over time or need to be exchanged or removed.

Minimum spend

£2,000–4,000.

Optimum age

Generally younger, twenties to thirties, as well as at the time of a facelift to give support to the lower face and neck. The better your bone structure, the longer your lift will last.

Ouch factor

2.

What is the alternative?

Adding fillers or fat to augment the chin and jaw area is a great alternative. It also enables you to try on the look to see if you like it, and then you can go for something more permanent.

EARS PINNED BACK

What it does

Unfortunately kids can be really cruel, and young children and teens are often teased about having prominent ears. Otoplasty is surgery to pin the ears closer to the head or to reduce the size and prominence of the ears.

The procedure

A sliver of cartilage may be removed from the back of the ear, and the remaining cartilage is stitched together so that it will appear closer to the head or the ear will be smaller in size. Surgery can also correct congenital deformities, as well as other cosmetic ear problems, to reshape the cartilage, or smooth out bits of cartilage that fold over the top of the ear.

Time in operating theatre

One to three hours.

Post-op effects and recovery time

You will have a pressure dressing placed around your head covering your ears. Your ears will feel tender, stiff and tight for a week, and you will be told to be careful not to disturb the ears and head bandages, which is harder for children than for adults. Bandages will be removed in five to ten days.

Risks

In addition to surgical risks, there can be asymmetries or irregularities in the ears, or raised scars. Numbness may last longer in some people.

How long it lasts

Permanent.

Minimum spend

£2,500–4,000.

Optimum age

Usually for children over the age of five, but also done on adults as needed.

Ouch factor

2.

What is the alternative?

Live with it, or keep your hair long.

FACE- AND NECKLIFT

Whenever one of my clients starts a conversation about facelifts with 'I don't expect to look 20 again,' my simple response is, 'Well, that's good, because you can't.' Even with a full facelift, it is not possible to make someone who is 50 look 25 again. That concept may have become confused with the male fantasy of trading in one 50-year-old wife for two 25-year-olds but sadly it does not work. While this may seem obvious, misconceptions about being able to turn the clock back in this fashion abound. But who really wants a Gen-X face anyway – unless someone can give you the body, teeth, hands, hair, energy and brain cells that go with being 25 again.

By the same token, a woman who has never had any work done by her fifth or sixth decade and is worried about looking like Joan Rivers if she goes for a lift now is being quite silly. Joan, by her own admission, is no stranger to cosmetic surgery. Is it sensible to think that a woman with jowls like Churchill and lines that could double for a road map could possibly come out looking like Joan after having one modestly done British-style facelift? I rest my case.

Ageing skin loses elasticity and develops wrinkles; fine lines or looseness cannot be entirely eliminated without pulling too tight, which would cause your mouth to go sideways, among other distortions. Some residual skin laxity even after a face- or necklift is not uncommon. In this case, your choices are to live with it, have something non-surgical to tighten up the neck without opening your scars or have a secondary surgery when you are ready. Consequently, the younger you are and the less dam-aged your skin is when you undergo surgery, the better result you can expect. However, that doesn't preclude you from having a home-run facelift at an older age. Having it early means you will see a less dramatic improvement. Having it later when everything has fallen means

WHAT IS THE VECTOR?

When doctors start talking about facial rejuvenation surgery, they speak about the vector they will use – which simply means the direction of the pull. For example, if you want your cheeks shifted up and out, this is called an oblique vector. If your mid-face is falling straight down, elevating it is considered a vertical vector. In many cases, you will need a combination of both vectors to get the job done properly. If the vectors are not well thought out, your face could go in the wrong direction. For example, a vertical vector fixes only the central portion. An oblique vector gives a more sideswept look, which can be good in some cases and overdone in others.

that your friends, family and possibly your butcher, dry cleaner and the cashier at your local WHSmith will know you've had something done to your face.

In general, rather than waiting until you look old and need surgery to make you look younger again you will have a better and more natural result when the signs of ageing are just beginning to appear but are not full blown. The end result is a refreshed appearance.

Facelifting has never been more complicated. There used to be a handful of commonly used techniques; now the possibilities are endless. The newest trend is to evaluate the face as a whole instead of individual segments of ageing.

What it does

A facelift is still the gold standard to correct a sagging, crêpey neck and jawline. It can tighten loose skin and muscle and remove or reposition excess fat to eliminate sagging. The most significant degree of improvement is usually seen in the jowls, lower face and neck. Facial shaping by removing, repositioning or adding soft tissue, rather than by tightening the skin and muscles alone, can offer a more harmonious result. It is important to understand what a facelift can and cannot do. A facelift or necklift takes care of sagging by removing excess skin, tightens the loose muscles underneath and elevates soft tissues. It does not treat lines and wrinkles, and it does not really address volume loss, unless fat or fillers are added. Some women will only have one facelift in their lifetime. It depends on when you start.

I had my first at 45, I will surely have at least one more in my lifetime and I wouldn't rule out a third. I had the 'short scar' variety, and as I wrote about my experience in *Financial Times How To Spend It* ('When a New Hairdo Just Won't Cut it Anymore', 15 September 2004), *Tatler* ('Can You Look Great After a Facelift – Without Friends

Guessing Why?, April 2005) and the magazine of the Oberoi Hotels & Resorts (the same year), the entire free world including all my exes must know about it by now.

> Having a facelift is like buying a car. It is brand new until you drive it out of the dealership, but from the moment your foot hits the pedal, the mileage starts piling up on you.

The procedure

Facelift surgery is performed under general anaesthetic in hospital. There is no one preferred method, and your surgeon should tailor his operation to your individual needs and goals. Although the actual facelift incisions vary, they generally start above the hairline at the temples and continue along a line in front of the ear or just inside the cartilage at the front of the ear, behind the earlobe and sometimes into the hairline. Another small incision is often made under the chin. Modified techniques may cut the scar in half, usually reducing the scar that extends behind the ear and avoiding altering the hairline, which makes a big difference to the patient. If you have spent your life making peace with your hair, as most women have, not having to change the way you wear it after having a lift is a huge deal. Your hairstylist will know you have had a little work done no matter what.

The surgeon separates the skin from the underlying fat and muscle. The underlying muscle fascia is tightened, along with the platysma muscle in the neck, and excess fat is removed. After the deep tissues are tightened, the excess skin is pulled up and back and then trimmed. The incisions are closed with stitches and/or staples on the scalp. In some cases, your face and neck may be wrapped in a gauzy turban or headband that is removed the next day, to minimise bruising and swelling. To drain any fluid that collects, a small tube may be inserted under the skin behind your ear for a day or two. Drains used to be placed routinely, but newer techniques are less bloody, and many surgeons now use them less often.

Plastic Makes Perfect

THE ART OF THE LIFT

Egad! Yikes! What kind of lift should you have? With all the clever names and acronyms out there, it is really hard to know for sure. Some procedures correct or improve most areas of the face and some were designed to enhance only specific sections. To further complicate matters, each surgeon has his own variations on all these themes, not to mention catchy names such as the 'Bandaid Lift' or 'Lifestyle Lift'.

Here are the top dozen lifts:

Conventional facelift Designed to lift sagging skin and the deeper structures. The incision lines are usually placed along or behind the hairline. Excess skin is excised, and facial skin, muscles and fat are resuspended in a higher position. This commonly includes the neck area, but not the brow or eyelids.

SMAS (Superficial (or Sub-) Muscular Aponeurotic System) lift The SMAS is responsible for your facial movements. Without it you would not be able to smile, frown, smirk or make other facial expressions. This area is lifted up and out, sort of diagonally. This can be done with the Platysma lift (necklift) as well.

Platysma lift (necklift, platysmaplasty) Often done in conjunction with a SMAS lift, this method targets sagging and loose skin of the neck and jowls. The platysma muscles are tightened and then sutured together down the middle, and hanging skin and excess fat is removed to give you a swan-like youthful neck.

S-lift Considered a modified approach in which the incision is made directly in front of the ear and the layers are moved and pulled laterally. The S-lift really only targets the lower third of the face; the upper face, eyelids and brow area are not significantly improved.

MACS lift (Minimal Access Cranial Suspension lift) Similar to an S-lift, with a bit of a twist. The incision is limited to where the skin meets the hairline above and in front of the ear, and is zigzag in shape so as to be easily concealed as hair grows around it. There is no extension behind the ear. A purse-string suture is used to yank up the cheeks, smooth the nasolabial folds and soften jowls (analogous to purse strings that close on top of a handbag; when a purse-string suture is placed in a circle and tightened, it elevates the tissue). It does not work brilliantly for the neck, but is ideal for younger women and men who don't need too much skin lifted or removed.

SOOF lift (Suborbicularis Oculi Fat lift) Intended to reposition the fat hiding deep under the eyelid muscles, in order to help correct a hollow or skeletal-looking under-eye area. Some surgeons include a cheeklift or mid-facelift as well.

Subperiosteal facelift Designed to lift the sub-orbital (below the eyes) area as well as the mid-face, a subperiosteal facelift provides a vertical lift to the soft tissues of the face. The suspension is accomplished by anchoring deep sutures directly to the edges of the temporalis fascia (connective tissue surrounding muscles) and tying them into place. It works on all the layers of tissue, down to the bone. For women in their late forties or fifties, an endoscopic subperiosteal approach can be combined with skin removal for best results in the lower third of the face.

Deep plane lift Performed in a deeper plane than a standard facelift, this procedure is like a SMAS lift with the nasolabial folds being improved by lifting the sagging fat pad that causes this fold. At the same time, this pad is repositioned upwards and backwards, improving cheekbone definition. There is a somewhat higher risk of nerve damage.

Temporal lift (lateral lift, lateral browlift) A more lateral-diagonal lift, this can also produce an exotic look on the outer arch of the brow. It can relieve folds and small wrinkles in the forehead, the glabella (between the brows) and crow's feet; it can also lift the cheek skin to restore a more chiselled look to the cheekbones where fat and loose skin have fallen south.

Mid-face lift Produces a refreshed look to sagginess around the under-eye, nasolabial, and upper mouth and outer upper lip area. One technique is done through an incision under the lower eyelid. This is a good option if you want or need a more vertical lift rather than a horizontal or diagonal windswept lift. The endoscopic mid-face technique requires two vertical incisions in the scalp slightly above the temples. The best candidates for pure endoscopic facial surgery are patients in their late thirties or early forties with good skin tone and early sagging of the brows and cheeks.

Mini-lift This is one of the great vagaries of cosmetic surgery; the term means different things to different doctors. Some surgeons consider a mini-lift to be a lateral lift with incisions placed only directly in front of the ears. This technique can improve the nasolabial folds but doesn't really do much for the neck. Others use the term to describe an upper facelift or lower facelift alone.

Time in operating theatre

Two to five hours, depending on the technique used and any other procedures done at the same time.

Post-op effects and recovery time

Contrary to what you might expect, a facelift does not cause you to double over in throbbing pain. There is some discomfort for a few days but severe pain is rare. You should rest for 72 hours, avoid placing added tension on the scars and sleep on your back. Cold compresses help reduce swelling and soothe pain. Most stitches are removed after five days. If staples are used in the scalp, they will come out after 10–14 days. Once dressings are off, you can shower and shampoo your hair – usually the next day. Some tightness and numbness is to be expected for a few weeks or longer. It is common to have lumps and bumps, and areas of hardness, especially around the cheeks, chin and neck, from swelling. Avoid alcohol, steam baths and saunas for several weeks, as these increase swelling. A facelift is a long process – don't expect to look or feel 100 per cent for at least a few weeks.

> **TISSUE GLUE**
>
> A neat little technique that can keep recovery, bleeding and scars to a minimum. Fibrin sealant, or fibrin 'glue', is a unique material that is often used during facelifts, breast procedures and large body techniques. The tissue glue or fibrin sealant is applied along the incision line. The sealant acts as a vasoconstrictor and closes off severed capillaries to literally seal the incision within a few minutes, so you don't need any sutures. See www.advancingbiosurgery.com.

Risks

Most post-op numbness is temporary. Poor or delayed healing and skin sloughing around the incisions are rare but may occur if there is too much tension on the skin, especially in smokers. A slight shift in the hairline is common, which is why informing your surgeon about how

Your Fabulous Face

109

you wear your hair is a good idea so that he can plan the incisions accordingly. Drains may be used to collect fluid or blood. Thickened or raised scars can be a problem. Injury to the nerves that control facial muscles is a potentially serious complication. Asymmetries or irregular contours are also possible.

How long it lasts

Results are permanent, and you will always look better for having had a facelift, although the ageing process marches on. You will need another one in five to ten years' time as your jawline starts to sag again.

Minimum spend

£5,000–10,000 and up, depending on the method used and the extent of the operation.

Optimum age

Typically forties and up, unless you live in LA, where any age goes.

Ouch factor

2 or 3, depending on the technique used.

What is the alternative?

For sagging skin, skin-tightening technologies can work to some degree. Endotine® or sutures (threads) with tiny cogs will hike up loose skin of the mid-face and jowls. Various volumising fillers, such as fat, Sculptra® and Restylane® Perlane, can produce a rejuvenating effect by plumping up cheeks and sunken areas. Liposuction of the neck may be an alternative for younger women with taut, elastic skin.

What's Up (or down) With Your Neck?

- **Low hanging glands**

  Your neck may look full before and even after a face- or necklift because of fatty bits, droopy skin, muscle bands or low-hanging glands. The submandibular gland (also called the mandibular or submaxillary gland) is a large salivary gland located below your mandible on each side of your jaw. In some cases, this gland can be tucked to clean up the neckline, but the procedure is somewhat controversial in plastic surgery circles. There are two camps: proponents who do it successfully on people who need it, and dissenters who don't think it should be undertaken. If you think you may be a candidate, seek out a highly experienced surgeon who has perfected the technique because when it is done poorly, irregularities may result that are hard to reverse.

- **Turkey wattle**

  If you have weakened or loose neck muscles, this may cause the appearance of vertical neck bands or muscle cords. To correct this, you may have a platysmaplasty. Incisions are made under your chin and/or behind your ears to access the neck muscle and place sutures to hold the tissue in place. Botox® can relax parts of the muscle temporarily.

- **Fat pouch**

  Liposuction can be used to remove the excess fat from the neck and jowls through tiny incisions made behind the ears or under the chin. A compression bandage is worn to reduce swelling and help skin contract. In some countries, fat dissolving injections have also been used to reduce the fat deposits in this area.

- **Jowly bits**

  If you have started to notice the formation of 'parentheses', or a divet on either side of your chin where fatty tissue can formed, you can have it streamlined with a filler. Restylane® Perlane, Evolence® or HydraFill® or another filler can be injected into this area to effectively smooth out your jawline.

- **Excess skin**

  Incisions are made behind the ear, and under the chin to perform a 'cervicoplasty' or lower facelift to trim away extra skin and lift the tissues back into place. Thermage® or Titan® may be performed to offer some skin-tightening effects.

Après the lift

Lifts work wonders in turning the clock back by about a decade or so, but they can't stop ageing forever. After spending a fortune on your face, you'll want to keep it looking its best to protect your investment for as long as possible.

- Botox® is the ideal treatment to maintain the effects of a forehead or browlift and eyelid procedures.
- A little tube of sunscreen is good insurance for your big investment. Think pale is the new tan! Choose a sunscreen with Avobenzone (Parsol® 1789), Zinc Oxide or Mexoryl® to protect skin from UVA and UVB rays. Go for an SPF of at least 15. Slather it on daily, and reapply every two hours to maintain a high level of protection throughout the day.
- Lifts do nothing for lines and skin texture. Forget the garden-variety facial and go for a peel, microdermabrasion and light therapy, which can improve the texture and quality of your skin.
- Quit smoking – smokers start to wrinkle and sag much sooner, and may need to go in for a touch-up after two years instead of five or more years.
- Take advantage of non-surgical treatments that can prolong the effects of your lift. Volumising fillers and skin-tightening devices are alternatives to more surgery when your jawline starts to square off again.

Patricia's turkey gobbler neck
Patricia had been saving to have her face done for five years, but

Plastic Makes Perfect

the timing was never right. She came to see me because her two-year-old granddaughter Philippa was sitting on her lap one day playing with the hanging skin on her neck. The toddler was literally poking at the wad of fat and flesh that had settled in her jowls. Patricia didn't know whether to laugh or cry. That was the impetus she needed to get going. She had her face lifted, and decided to go for the upper eyes too. Philippa has moved on to play with a Tinky Winky doll, since there is nothing to tug at on Granny's neck any more.

NIP TIP
Wrinkles are like cracks; creases are like grooves; folds are like tunnels. When they turn up, they need to be filled, but each in a different way and with a different substance.

SURGERY BLUNDERS

Results of cosmetic surgery can be unpredictable, and sometimes things can go pear-shaped. Many complications are due to the healing process or the failure of the surgeon to recognise pre-existing conditions that have caused the problem.

Pulled face/lateral sweep

Symptoms

Droopiness of the central portion of the face; too much tension along the jawline.

Solutions

Mid-face lift procedure can elevate the cheeks and reposition the cheek muscle; fat and fillers will fill in and create a cushion between the bone and the skin.

Your Fabulous Face

113

Nerve damage

Symptoms

Weakness of the nerves that are responsible for the movement of the face or the nerves that supply sensation to the face and neck; inability to close the eyes or droopiness of the cheek, mouth or lips.

Solutions

The majority of nerve damage is only temporary and recovers on its own within a few months. Botox® injections may be used to weaken the stronger muscle while the nerve heals itself.

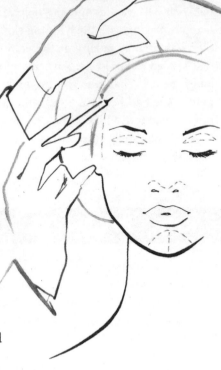

Earlobe pull

Symptoms

Excessive tugging on the earlobe from the tightened skin after a facelift or necklift may create an unnatural look around the ears, which is sometimes referred to as 'pixie ears' or 'devil's ears' because of the ears' pointy appearance.

Solutions

Separating the earlobe from the cheek and then recreating the natural, curved appearance of the earlobe can repair the pulled earlobe.

Under-eye hollows

Symptoms

Removing eyelid fat can create a hollow or sunken area around the eye, leaving a sad or skeletonised look.

Solutions

Restoring fullness with a filler or fat levels out the depression.

Pulled-down eyelids

Symptoms

Under-eye incisions can cause scar contraction that pulls the lower lid down, resulting in the whites of the eyes (sclera) being more visible. This in turn can create irritation from eye exposure, redness and dry eye syndrome.

Solutions

Insertion into the lower eyelid of a graft from your own hard palate (roof of the mouth) can raise the lid to a more normal position. Sometimes a mid-face lift can help if the cheeks have descended and are pulling further on the lower eyelid.

Eyelids that don't close

Symptoms

Too much skin and/or muscle removed from the upper eyelids can cause incomplete eyelid closure (lagopthalmos), as well as dry eye, reflexive tearing, burning and a sensation of sand in the eye.

Solutions

Insertion of a weight in the upper eyelid will sometimes pull down the lid so that it can close sufficiently. A surgical repair may also be done by placing a skin graft into the upper lid.

Hairline pulled back

Symptoms

Wide appearance to the temporal region or an unnaturally high fore-head, with an unnaturally pulled-back hairline.

Solutions

Hair transplants can fill in the hairline; surgery with an incision placed at the hairline can pull it down into a better position.

NOSE RESHAPING

What it does

Rhinoplasty can correct the obvious cosmetic issues of how the nose looks and whether it is in proportion to the other facial features, as well as functional problems including breathing obstructions and problems arising from traumatic injuries. It is usually recommended to wait until the age of 14 for girls and 16 for boys (girls mature sooner). The nose may not be fully developed at a younger age. The most common reasons for rhinoplasty are: a nose that is crooked, too large or too wide for the face, a bump on the bridge, a profile that is out of proportion, a droopy or thick tip and flared nostrils. As you age, the supportive structures of the nose diminish, and the shape and position will ultimately change. The nose may appear longer and the tip eventually comes down. Rhinoplasty is not just about making the nose smaller any more. Some noses need to be lengthened, augmented or narrowed for the best look. You can have a natural-looking nasal correction, instead of the very obvious 'nose job' look of yesteryear. Previous nasal surgery may also be corrected by a second operation, so you don't have to live with a nose you don't like.

The procedure

Rhinoplasty is usually performed under general anaesthetic and incisions are sometimes made inside the rim of the nostrils. In some cases, tiny, inconspicuous incisions are also made on the rim of the nose to reduce the width of the nostrils. An open technique is used if a more complex correction is needed or for a secondary rhinoplasty procedure. A small incision is made outside the nose across the columella (the strip of skin that divides your nostrils). The outer tissue of the nose can be turned back, providing visualisation of the structures inside. There will be an incision at the base of the nose that may be V-, U- or Z-shaped to camouflage it. In a closed rhinoplasty, the incisions are made inside the nose so that there is no visible scar. Soft tissues of the nose are separated from the underlying structures, and the cartilage and bone are reshaped. If your nose is reduced in size, the nasal bones may be fractured. If your nose needs to be built up in certain areas, grafts of nasal cartilage, ear cartilage, rib cartilage and bone may be used. The skin and soft tissues will shrink to fit the bony architecture of your new nasal shape. Breathing problems may be corrected by reducing obstructions and improving the airway. A splint may be placed on the bridge of the nose to hold the tissues in place and to protect the nose.

Time in operating theatre

One to three hours.

Post-op effects and recovery time

A splint will generally be applied for five to seven days. The nose may be packed lightly with gauze that will be removed in one to two days. You will be instructed not to get the splint or tape wet. Internal stitches

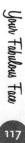

are self-absorbing, so they will not require removal. You may have bleeding from the nose, and you will have to change your gauze bandages, as they will get soiled. By the end of the first week, splints, bandages and external sutures will be removed. There will be swelling, pressure and stuffiness for several weeks. If the nasal bones are fractured, you may have bruising around the eyelid area or bloodshot eyes. Be careful about blowing your nose, as doing so can cause bleeding. Avoid contact sports or any activity that may risk injury to the nose for four to six weeks. The nose will remain very tender at this stage, and if you bang it accidentally, you will see stars. Eyeglasses will have to be taped to the forehead, off the bridge of the nose, for the first several weeks as the bone sets. Your nose may be numb, and the swelling will take longest to settle down in the tip – it can take 6 to 12 months. The thicker your skin, the longer it may take to see the final shape in the tip. If your nose seems very swollen for a long time, your doctor may be able to inject the tip with a little bit of steroid to speed up settling.

Risks

Bleeding is common after rhinoplasty. There is no such thing as a perfect nose and it is not uncommon for a correction to be required or requested after the nose has settled into its new shape. Some irregularities of cartilage and bone are to be expected and are present in all noses. Secondary nasal surgery will usually not be done for at least 6 to 12 months, until the tissues have fully healed and all the swelling has gone down.

How long it lasts

Results are permanent, although with age, the tip of the nose will drop become thicker and seem to look bigger in proportion to your deflating cheeks.

Minimum spend

£4,000–6,000; more for revisions and re-dos.

Optimum age

Generally younger – late teens, twenties and thirties; but it is not uncommon to have your nose refined later in life or at the time of a facelift.

Ouch factor

2.

What is the alternative?

Fillers can be used to fill out any subtle defects in the nose.

> ### Mona and her mother
> Mona was 27 when she decided to get her nose done. Coming from a very traditional family, she felt nervous and wanted to do it in secret. She assumed that she could just show up at her parents' house one night for dinner and no one would know. Of course, reality set in when I explained that her mother would surely be able to tell that her eldest daughter's nose had been altered, and it would be better to involve her in the process from the beginning. There is something about having your mother change your dressing and bring you a cup of tea that is very comforting. Mona's mother was actually delighted when she approached her – and would have been really cross if Mona had tried to hide it from her. She also confessed that she had hers done before she got married and never told Mona's father about it!

Ask The Beauty Junkie®

Is there any way to eliminate the baggy skin on top of the eyes without surgery?
Excess skin of the upper or lower eyelids has to be removed to be eliminated, which requires a surgical procedure called blepharoplasty. A browlift may also be recommended in addition to or instead of eyelid surgery to raise the eyebrows, if they contribute to fullness of the upper lids. Lasers and peels can soften lines and Botox® is great for crow's feet, but these will not relieve the excess skin.

Can your nose be operated on more than once?
In fact, it is more common than you may think to have a rhinoplasty two, three or more times. Nasal surgery can be quite tricky and since the nose is the central feature of the face, it is subject to a lot of scrutiny by its owner and onlookers alike. It is also more difficult to correct a previous rhinoplasty than other cosmetic procedures, as there is usually more scar tissue and the results are less predictable.

What is the ideal age to have a facelift?
There is really no ideal age – it varies from person to person. However, the trend is to do it early, before you really need it and your neck starts to slide down into your chest. Women who have their first lift in their forties tend to look really good in their fifties. The average age today for women is late forties to mid-fifties. For men, it is about five to ten years later.

After a facelift, will everything just fall down again after even more five or ten years?
This is a big misconception. A facelift turns back the clock, but it neither stops it completely nor accelerates it. Your face doesn't suddenly fall after a facelift so that you look worse, or older. In fact, you will always look better because you had a facelift than if you never had had one.

Plastic Makes Perfect

Is there such a thing as a 'non-surgical' facelift?
A non-surgical facelift is a misnomer. Although there are several techniques being used to approximate some of the effects of a facelift, these are not substitutes for a proper surgical facelift. Among these methods are fat transfer, Sculpta® and other volume plumpers; and Thermage® and other skin-tightening devices. These techniques may offer some improvement along the lines of what a facelift can offer; however, the end result is minimal in comparison to surgery.

7

Your Beautiful Breasts and Upper Half

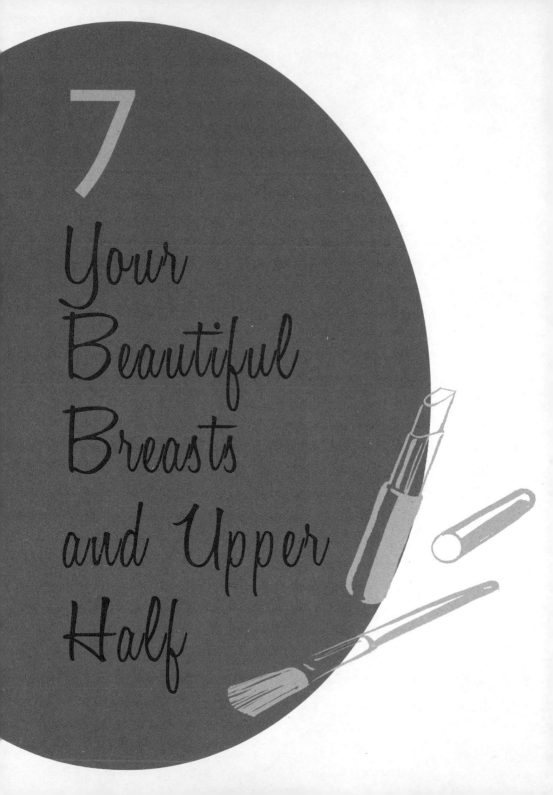

The moment of truth may come in a department store fitting room, or when faced with your naked body in the mirror. At some point in every woman's life she will look at her own breasts and wonder 'what if?'. Whether they are too big, too small, droopy or flat, no one can overestimate the effect a woman's breasts have on her overall self-esteem; some women are clearly defined by their breasts from a very early age. Your once perky, firm breasts inevitably become floppy and soft somewhere along the line.

BREAST AUGMENTATION

Breasts are like snowflakes: no two are exactly alike. Although it may seem like a simple operation to the novice, the procedure is actually very complex and creating great breasts is truly an art form, requiring a surgeon with both a keen aesthetic eye and good judgement. Breast reshaping is not all about volume. It is more about proportion and dimension.

What it does

Breast implants are used to increase breast fullness for women with modest breasts, or to replace volume for women who have lost it after pregnancies, breastfeeding or weight loss. There is an endless variety of implant designs, shapes, sizes and

SIZE COUNTS

Doctors don't think about breasts in terms of cup sizes (B, C, D, etc.); they think in cubic centimetres (cc). If you are flat-chested, even a small implant will seem big to you at first. It's all about proportions and measurements. For example, a 350cc implant on a size 6 girl with a small frame will look quite different to the same-size implant on a woman who wears a size 12 and has broad shoulders. To try on a size and see how it looks, fill two plastic bags with salt, rice or something soft and mouldable, and stuff them into a bra in the size you are considering.

BETTER SHAPE WITHOUT THE STUFFED LOOK

This new era of breast enhancement allows women to take charge of their breast augmentation desires, goals and mission. If you want your breasts to have a better shape, prettier nipples, softer volume, the choices are yours now. Breast augmentation is not just about making them bigger anymore – you can literally change the shape and keep the size you want to be, or used to have.

textures, all of which have advantages and disadvantages. A breast implant is basically a soft, silicone envelope with any one of various fillers that is surgically implanted under the tissues of your chest to simulate natural breast tissue. The sac may be filled with a silicone gel or saline (salt water). The implants can be round or teardrop-shaped, with a textured or smooth coating. Cohesive gel silicone implants are thicker and firmer, so they last longer, virtually eliminate the risks of leakage or rupture, and offer the best shape and projection.

The procedure

Performed under general anaesthetic, surgery consists of making an incision, lifting the breast tissue, creating a pocket in the breast area and placing an envelope containing a soft implant material underneath. An incision may be made in any one of these places: the crease below your breast, around the areola, under your armpit or through the tummy button, which is less common. If you want to keep your implants a secret, a scar directly on the breast can give you away. Implants can be placed either under the chest muscle or directly under the breast tissue.

Risks

Some common risks associated with breast implants:

- Rippling, indentations
- Implant failure
- Hardening due to scar tissue

- Temporary or permanent loss of sensation
- Formation of calcium deposits in surrounding tissue
- Implant shifting.

General complications include bleeding, blood clot and skin loss resulting from insufficient blood flow to the skin. Capsular contracture can cause painful hardening of the breast or distort its appearance. Depending on your age when you have implants, you will most likely replace them in your lifetime. It is impossible to predict how long individual implants will last, but they can be very durable. They can be removed at any time. If you have had them for many years, removing them may – depending on their size and your skin quality – leave you drooping. In this case, a breastlift may be recommended.

Time in operating theatre

One to two hours.

Post-op effects and recovery time

Your chest will be wrapped with gauze bandage as well as a surgical bra or elastic band for additional protection and support. You may also have drainage tubes placed in the incision for several days to help eliminate excess fluid. After five to seven days, the gauze dressing will be removed and you will wear a non-underwire support or sports bra continuously for several weeks. Your breasts will be taped high on your chest, and will feel firm and swollen. As the swelling goes down, they will drop into a more normal position and shape. You will have to minimise arm movements and bend from the knees only. You will heal more quickly if you avoid stretching and lifting, in order to prevent the separation of the muscle and tissue surrounding the implants. You may be able to resume work within a week, but avoid aerobic activity until soreness subsides. The scars will remain pink for several months.

Your Beautiful Breasts and Upper Half

How long it lasts

Breasts will droop with gravity, ageing and weight loss. The average lifespan of a breast implant is 16 years.

Minimum spend

£4,000–7,000.

Optimum age

Twenties to thirties, post-childbirth or at a later age.

Ouch factor

3.

THE IMPLANTS ARE COMING

Although Allergan and Mentor are widely accepted as the premier implant manufacturers worldwide. Here are some other brands on the market:

- www.breastimplantstoday.com
- www.mentor4me.com
- www.sientra.com
- www.implantspip.com
- www.eurosilicone.com
- www.nagor.co.uk
- www.smart-plant.com

What is the alternative?

If you want higher, fuller breasts, a breastlift without implants may be a possible option. In the not-too-distant future Macrolane® may be available to enhance the breast by the implantation of hyaluronic acid gel. Fat is also being used by some surgeons to replace lost breast volume.

Thanks for the mammaries

It will come as no surprise to anyone walking down a high street that breast augmentation is the most popular cosmetic surgery in Britain. But Playmate of the Month enhanced breasts are so yesterday. Women who seek breast augmentation today are just like you and me. They may have breastfed a few children and just want some volume back, or they are tired of having to wear water bras that spring a leak in order to get some cleavage. They may also feel that their upper body is not in proportion to their lower body.

Saline-filled implants are still around if that is your preference, but silicone gel is the most used implant worldwide. The newest variety, called cohesive gel, has been available in Europe since 1995. The name indicates that the gel is thicker and stronger than earlier formulations, so it has little or no chance of leakage or rupture. If you cut into an older gel implant, the liquid-like silicone will escape from the implant shell. When you slice open a cohesive gel implant, the implant will maintain its shape. These are called form stable implants and they are like a Rowntrees™ fruit gum. The advantages are better shape, less wrinkling, and a softer and more natural feel. There are

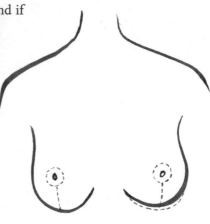

more choices available in height, width and sizes to customise the surgery so that you can have the best breasts for your frame. Another innovation, called Soft Touch Cohesive Gel™, combines softer cohesive with high-cohesive gel for a more individualised look and perkier nipples that stand to attention.

If silicone has you worried, remember that silicone has been used safely in the body for ages in other medical devices such as pacemakers and heart valves. All breast implants have a silicone

Your Beautiful Breasts and Upper Half

elastomer shell; it is what they are filled with that makes the difference. After 14 long years, in 2006 the US FDA (Food and Drug Administration) finally gave approval for silicone gel implants to be brought back to market. The FDA is recommending a follow-up MRI (Magnetic Resonant Imaging) two years post breast augmentation and every three years thereafter to discover possible implant rupture, although most doctors do not think that this is needed. The decision to bring silicone back is making thousands of women (and their surgeons) very happy indeed.

BIGGER BREASTS – THE NATURAL WAY

Want fuller, rounder and higher breasts that are technically all yours? Auto-augmentation is a method of enhancing your breasts using your own breast tissue, bypassing the need for implants. The surgeon performs a breastlift to tighten up the breast skin, and uses your own glands to add volume, shape and some perk to your posture.

NIP TIP

Consider having a baseline mammogram before breast surgery, depending on your age and family history of breast cancer, particularly on your mother's side. In America, mammograms are recommended for women over 40. The NHS breast-screening programme is for women between 50 and 70. However, you can have a mammogram privately if you so desire.

BREASTLIFT

Perky breasts are a fleeting concept. When you are young, you don't quite appreciate them. When you hit 40, you just hope they are still self-supporting. Most women have what I call 'working breasts'. They are not just there to fill up a 36C bra and attract attention in a plunging neckline: they are a food source. So after you have finished breastfeeding a few babies, it seems only fair that you take them in for a tune-up.

What it does

A breastlift raises and reshapes breasts that have sagged as a result of pregnancy, breastfeeding and the natural forces of gravity.

Asymmetries can also be evened out. These are actually very common: about 80 per cent of women will have some difference between her breasts. A breastlift can also reduce the size of the areola, the darker skin surrounding the nipple. If your nipples have expanded from breastfeeding, an incision placed around the nipple areola complex will reduce and reshape them. A breastlift can be combined with an implant when volume needs to be enhanced. If cleavage is the goal, an implant is often essential. The operation reshapes your existing breast tissue, reduces excess skin and moves your nipples to a higher position. If your breasts are very saggy, adding a bigger implant to fill them up will only make matters worse. Think rock in a sock.

The procedure

Breastlift surgery is performed under general anaesthetic in hospital. Several techniques can be used, depending on the degree of sagging. Surgery consists of removing excess skin from around the areola, and possibly also from the bottom of the breast, with shifting of the breast skin to tighten the skin envelope, and smoothing of the skin to elevate the nipple and areola to their original position. Specific breastlifts fall into the more traditional incision pattern and modified or scar-saving techniques,

> **Take the Pencil Test:** Place a pencil in the fold under the breast where your breast meets your chest wall. If the pencil does not fall, you have failed the pencil test, which indicates that you are drooping. Another version of the pencil test is to stick a pencil vertically into your cleavage while wearing a bra. If the pencil doesn't fall, you have passed the test and your cleavage is good as gold!

which have gained popularity in the last decade. The traditional anchor incision involves incisions made around the nipple areola complex, vertically on the breast and horizontally under the breast. The more tissue that needs to be removed, the longer the scar, but the more shaping is possible. The vertical mastopexy, also called a lollipop, ice-cream-cone or LeJeur technique, falls somewhere in between the traditional and minimal scar technique, and is widely suitable for many types of breasts. The donut mastopexy, which involves an incision

Your Beautiful Breasts and Upper Half

placed only around the areola, is usually reserved for women with small breasts that are only mildly droopy where very little skin needs to be removed. Most women need more than just this incision to sufficiently lift their breasts and create a nice shape.

Time in operating theatre

Two to five hours.

Post-op effects and recovery time

You will leave the hospital with an elastic bandage or a surgical bra over gauze dressings. Your breasts will be tender and swollen for several days. Within a few days, a soft support bra will replace the bandages or you will wear a surgical bra constantly for several weeks over a layer of gauze. Stitches will be removed after five to twelve days. Avoid lifting anything over your head or engaging in strenuous sports for three to four weeks. Some loss of feeling in your nipples and breast skin can occur, caused by post-operative swelling. Sensation usually returns as the swelling subsides over four to six weeks.

Risks

Bleeding and infection are rare, but can cause scars to widen. It is possible to have unevenly positioned nipples, permanent loss of sensation and breast asymmetry. Perhaps the biggest risk is your acceptance of the scars, which can remain raised and red for months, and then gradually fade. If breastfeeding is a consideration, make sure this is reviewed in detail before going ahead with surgery. You may not be able to breastfeed after a lift, as the incision may interfere with milk ducts.

How long it lasts

Results are long lasting; however, breasts will continue to sag with age and weight changes, or future pregnancies.

Minimum spend

£4,000–6,000; more with implants.

Optimum age

Usually done when you have finished having children, after major weight loss or if you have a breast asymmetry; any age from 18 up.

Ouch factor

3.

What is the alternative?

If your breasts are petite, placing an implant may give you enough lift, without having any skin removed. If you have just a small amount of wobbly skin, skin-tightening devices such as Thermage® might give you some spring back.

Angela's extra lines

Angela was newly single after her partner of 12 years left her for his much younger secretary (how original!). Getting undressed in front of a new man was something she dreaded, so she decided to have her breasts lifted to regain her confidence and feel sexy naked again. She had been a 36C at one time, but now in her mid-forties, she was more like a droopy 36D. Her goal was to have a small lift to keep the size but make the girls perky again. The surgeon told her that he would use the LeJeur technique (named after Belgian plastic surgeon Madeleine LeJeur), which involved a scar around her nipples and one vertical line running down each breast. Angela agreed and signed up. When she went to see her surgeon after surgery, she hadn't yet seen her new breasts under the dressings. The nurse removed them, and much to Angela's surprise, she had scars she was not expecting. She demanded to see the surgeon and said, 'You never told me I would have lines under my breasts!' His steely response was, 'I did what I thought was best.' Angela was in shock – but there was nothing she could do. The ropey-looking scars all the way under each breast were way more than she had signed on for. She couldn't wear low-cut tops or halters because the ends of her scars almost reached into her armpits. Sadly, for the first year, those scars made her more self-conscious than her saggy 36D chest had.

BREAST REDUCTION

Although for some women having large breasts may seem a dream come true, if yours are a 38EE, you may not be all that happy to carry them around. Heavy, hanging breasts can become a major burden and prevent you from enjoying sports, buying good clothes and feeling comfortable with yourself.

What it does

Breast reduction can remedy any number of concerns, from emotional pain and physical pain in the neck and back caused by large breasts to asymmetries in size or shape.

The procedure

The traditional method involves an anchor-shaped incision that circles the areola, extends downwards and follows the natural curve of the crease beneath the breast. The surgeon removes excess glandular tissue, fat and skin, and moves the nipple and areola into their new position. The skin is then brought from both sides of the breast down and around the areola, shaping the new contour of the breast. In most cases, the nipples remain attached to their blood vessels and nerves. However, if your breasts are very large and dangling, the nipples may have to be completely removed and grafted into a higher position, which can result in a loss of sensation. Stitches are usually located around the areola, in a vertical line extending downwards and along the lower crease of the breast. Other techniques eliminate the horizontal portion of the scar

Plastic Makes Perfect

entirely, so that the scars are only around the nipple and vertical. A J- or L-shape pattern can also be used to avoid a longer scar under the breast.

Time in operating theatre

Two to five hours.

Post-op effects and recovery time

After surgery, you'll be wrapped in an elastic bandage or a surgical bra over gauze dressings. A drain may be placed in each breast for the first few days. The bandages will be removed a day or two after surgery, and you will continue to wear the surgical bra around the clock for several weeks. Stitches will be removed in one to two weeks. Your first menstruation following surgery may cause your breasts to swell and hurt. You may also experience random, shooting pains for a few weeks, especially when you move around or cough. Expect some loss of feeling in your nipples and breast skin, caused by the swelling. This should fade over the next six weeks; in some cases, however, it may last longer, and occasionally it may be permanent. Although you may be up and about in a few days, your breasts will be sore. Limit exercise to stretching, bending and swimming until your energy level returns. You'll need a good athletic bra for support. No sex for two weeks, since arousal can cause swelling, and avoid anything but gentle contact with your new breasts for about six weeks. Some crusting and fluid draining from your incisions is normal. It will take six months until your breasts fully settle into their new size and shape.

Risks

Breast reduction is not a simple operation, and there is always the possibility of complications. You can develop small sores around your nipples after surgery that can be treated with antibiotic creams. The scars are extensive and permanent. They often remain lumpy and red for months, before gradually fading. You may also have slightly mismatched breasts or unevenly positioned nipples, or nipples that are too large. Breastfeeding may not be possible, since the surgery removes many of the milk ducts leading to the nipples. You may also have permanent loss of feeling in your nipples or breasts. Rarely, the nipple and areola may lose their blood supply and the tissue will die.

NIP TIP
If it goes wrong the first time round, don't go back for more punishment, even if correction is offered for free. Get a second opinion, and consider getting a new doctor or clinic to put it right.

How long it lasts

Breast size and shape will change with future pregnancies, hormonal shifts, weight fluctuations, age and going braless too often.

Minimum spend

£4,000–7,000.

Optimum age

For women over the age of 18 who have finished developing naturally; women who are not planning to breastfeed and have finished having children.

Ouch factor

3.

What is the alternative?

If your breasts have a lot of fatty tissue, liposuction alone can reduce breast size, leaving minimal scars. Liposuction can also remove excess fat from the armpit area.

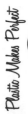

BREAST RECONSTRUCTION

'It's C-A-N-C-E-R.' Thump, your heart skips a beat. The fear of diagnosis and treatment are compounded by the fear of losing a breast, and with it, your femininity, attractiveness and identity. Finding out about breast reconstruction should begin when you first hear the 'C' word, so that you don't make hasty decisions that might limit your future options.

I have a special place in my heart for breast cancer survivors. They are some of the most courageous and impressive women I know. If you are battling the disease, these are some of the best resources to educate yourself about your treatment and reconstruction options:

- www.cancerandcareers.org
- www.cancerbackup.org.uk
- www.breastcancercare.org.uk
- www.breastcancer.org.

What it does

Designed to improve congenital breast deformities and for women who have undergone a lumpectomy or mastectomy, breast reconstruction takes a variety of forms. It may be performed immediately after a mastectomy, or it can be delayed for weeks or years. Immediate reconstruction can involve the placement of an implant or tissue expander that will eventually be replaced by an implant. When reconstruction is performed by an expert surgeon, it can beautifully restore your breasts to looking very natural.

The procedure

Breasts can be reconstructed using an implant, your own tissue or a combination of both. It is usually not a one-time operation. Following the first surgery, the doctor may need to replace a tissue expander, insert an implant, or perform nipple and areola reconstruction. Cosmetic work on the other breast may be done at the same time so that your breasts will appear symmetrical and identical.

Skin expansion After the mastectomy, if your skin is very tight you may need tissue expansion prior to reconstruction. A balloon expander is placed under the skin and chest muscle, and is gradually filled with salt-water solution to stretch the skin. The process will take several weeks to a few months, at which point either the expander will be left in or a permanent implant will be placed, and the areola can be reconstructed.

Flap reconstruction This method grafts your own tissue (generally from the torso area) to create a skin flap. The surgery involves reconnecting blood vessels contained in the tissue to the grafting site. The advantage of this surgery is that your own skin is used, but it is more complex and involves considerable scarring and recovery, since there are two surgical sites that have to heal.

Time in operating theatre

Two to five hours, depending on the procedure.

Post-op effects and recovery time

You will be tired and sore. You may need to wear a drain for between one and two weeks to make sure your body expels all excess fluid. After a week to ten days, the stitches will be removed. Recovery time may be up to six weeks, but it will vary depending on the extent of surgery. For three to six weeks you will need to avoid unnecessary stretching, lifting and any intense physical activity, including sex. Although you will not feel sensation as you would in your normal breast, you may begin to feel something over time.

Risks

Capsular contracture is the most common risk. This involves a hardening of the breast caused by tightening of the scar surrounding the implant. Rarely, patients experience bleeding, fluid collection, infection of the implant (which requires removal), excessive scar tissue or difficulties with anaesthesia. While there is no evidence that surgery will either prevent future cancer or cause it to return, continue to visit your doctor for regular mammograms to keep your new breasts healthy. Breast reconstruction and implants have no known effect on chemotherapy, but it is important to notify the radiologist who performs your mammogram of your surgical history, particularly if you had reconstruction with an implant.

How long it lasts

Results are permanent.

Minimum spend

£5,000–10,000; in some cases, may be covered by private health insurance or the NHS.

Optimum age

When you have undergone mastectomy to eliminate any remnant of cancer; age is not a determining factor.

Ouch factor

3.

What is the alternative?

External breast forms made from foam, silicone and cotton can be worn inside your bra.

> ### Brenda beats breast cancer
> Brenda struggled with hefty 36DD breasts. It was the overwhelming fear of surgery and pain that stopped her from having them reduced. One day she discovered a lump in the shower and was terrified. Her gynaecologist referred her to an oncologic surgeon next door to her office, who told her that it was cancer and both breasts would have to go. She was not even given the option of reconstruction. Brenda called my office and begged for an appointment straight away, but I was at a medical conference abroad. My office gave her my mobile number as she was almost hysterical. I advised her to see a plastic surgeon to see what all her options were before making any decisions. Fortunately, she discovered the cancer early, so her options were very favourable. After seeing two plastic surgeons, she arranged to have immediate reconstruction with a tissue expander on only one breast (not both, as the previous surgeon had advised). Although the experience was hard for Brenda and her family, her final result was a nicely reconstructed breast on one side and a reduction procedure in her normal,

healthy breast to restore symmetry. For Brenda, breast cancer was not a death sentence.

ARMLIFT

What it does

An armlift, or brachioplasty, is an operation to remove loose, flabby skin and fat that can give upper arms the dreaded nicknames bingo wings, bat wings and dinner lady arms. Liposuction can be combined with this procedure to give the arms a firmer appearance and shapelier look. It can also clean up those annoying and unsightly rolls of fat that always seem to be trying to escape from under your bra.

The procedure

The surgical approach depends on the droopiness of your skin. Incisions will be made along the inner arm from the elbow to the axilla (armpit), where the scars are best hidden. After surgery, excess fluid will be drained from the body through a rubber tube. A modified technique that involves placing the scar just into the armpit is also used. Results will not be as successful as with the traditional procedure, but a modified armlift can be a compromise if you have slightly slack arms with good skin tone.

Time in operating theatre

Two to four hours.

Post-op effects and recovery time

Recovery will take one to two weeks. You will be able to return to work within about two weeks but should avoid heavy lifting. It is important to protect the area of incision after surgery to ensure proper healing and to continue wearing dressings with elastic support. It is also important to elevate your arms with pillows for maximum comfort.

This operation is not for the squeamish and is a zero-fun procedure. There is a big trade-off between sculpted arms and a long scar that could preclude you from going strapless or showing off your results.

Risks

Visible scars are a major concern. Other possible complications include persistent swelling, bruising, numbness and change in feeling caused by nerve injury. If you have previously had a mastectomy or surgery for lymph nodes under the arms, or if you have frequent sweat gland infections, your doctor will have to determine if you are a good candidate for an armlift.

How long it lasts

Long-term results, although upper arms will start to sag again.

Minimum spend

£3,500–5,000.

Optimum age

Usually reserved for women who have lost a few stone, or as a last resort when nothing else will work.

Ouch factor

3.

What is the alternative?

Skin-tightening devices such as Thermage® and Titan®, as well as non-invasive fat busters, can be used for the arms. Liposuction alone is not ideal if your skin is loose and saggy. Religious weightlifting can help up to a point.

Ask The Beauty Junkie®

At what age can you have breast enlargement?
Generally, plastic surgeons prefer to wait at least until a girl has stopped growing (the FDA's recent approval of silicone gel implants was for breast augmentation in women aged 22 and older). Teens should not be rushing to have breast implants. This decision has long-term consequences and must be considered carefully. Parental involvement is critical, as no surgeon can operate on a minor without parental consent.

If am not sure about having more children, is it better to postpone having a breast reduction until I have finished having kids?
If being able to breastfeed is important to you, wait until you are done with having children to have incisional breast surgery. Future pregnancies will stretch your breast tissue all over again.

What is capsular contracture?
Scar tissue forms around all implanted materials as a natural part of the healing process. Scar tissue around a breast implant is not troublesome unless it tightens. An abnormally tight scar is known as a capsular contracture.

What can I do if I don't scar well?
If you have a history of bad scarring or thickened scars such as keloids, or delayed healing from past surgical procedures, inform your physician before having surgery. In general, the immediate scars will remain somewhat thickened and red for weeks and often months, then gradually become less obvious, ideally eventually fading to thin lines. If your scars do not heal well, they can be revised with additional surgery, injections of steroids, silicone gel patches or laser resurfacing.

What can be done about inverted nipples?
Inverted nipples may have a hole or a flat, slit or depressed appearance. There is often a lack of tissue that gives the nipple an

Plastic Makes Perfect

indented appearance. Corrective surgery is more of a cosmetic than a medical necessity, but it is best to wait until you have finished breastfeeding and do not intend to do so in the future, as the operation often involves severing the milk ducts. Another way to improve inverted nipples is to inject a filler, such as Radiesse®, to add projection so that the nipple looks normal.

Can breast implants really look natural?
In a word, yes! The typical client I see today for breast augmentation is just like you or me. She may have had her children, or lost some weight, or never had much of a chest since puberty. Not every woman who goes in for breast implants wants to look like the stereotypical bimbo. With today's naturally shaped implants and superior silicone fillers, a natural look is actually quite achievable. It's all about having good communication with a plastic surgeon and knowing what you want and what your anatomy will allow. The other secret to looking natural is to choose a smaller implant rather than something in the melon or soccer ball-size category. Breasts do not usually sit high up on your chest, so be wary when you are asking for more cleavage, that this is may end up being a more obviously enhanced look.

8

Your Lovely Lower Half

Your shape from the waist down has a lot to do with genetics and, of course, hormones. Every woman is born with a certain body type, and develops different levels of body fat and muscle mass. Your body type is completely determined by at least one of your parents and is often very hard to change on your own.

WHAT IS YOUR BODY TYPE?

Endomorphs Tend to have bigger bones, round faces, larger thighs and hips; stocky with a high waist and higher levels of body fat.
Mesomorphs Athletic build; hourglass or ruler shape; broad shoulders and a narrow waist.
Ectomorphs Thin, linear appearance; narrow waist, hips, and shoulders; low levels of body fat.

WHAT IS YOUR BODY SHAPE?

Hourglass Well-proportioned upper and lower body; narrow waist; a tendency to gain weight mostly in hips and chest area.
Pear Larger lower body, smaller upper body; a tendency to carry weight below the waist.
Apple Bigger on the top half than on the bottom half; slim hips and a large chest and stomach.
Ruler Reed-like and slim; long and lean; less contrast between the size of hips, waists and shoulders.

But if you didn't win the gene pool lottery, don't despair. With some self-discipline and a little help from a cosmetic surgeon, you can seriously improve the shape you were dealt.

Your Lovely Lower Half

For the past decade, liposuction has seemed like the Holy Grail for anyone who wants to change her shape. It has been the most popular cosmetic surgical procedure worldwide, for obvious reasons. Who doesn't have some fat she would like to get rid of?

Whereas dieting reduces your weight and size all over, liposuction reduces the overall number of your fat cells, and has the ability to change your figure flaws and contours. It is a safe and effective way to remove bulges from almost any area. Another advantage of liposuction is that you don't burn any bridges. You can always go back and have skin surgery later.

What it does

Stubborn fat deposits (such as saddlebags and on knees) that are hard to get rid of by cutting carbs and jogging around Hyde Park are ideal targets for liposuction. Most body parts can be suctioned – from your neck down to your ankles. The best areas for women are the abdomen, inner thighs, outer thighs, hips, flanks and knees. Liposuction can even be used to reduce heavy breasts. Evaluate your body in distinct units (the upper abdomen, lower abdomen, knees, etc.) and prioritise the areas that would benefit most from recontouring. If you are quite large, you may have to undergo these procedures in stages. Liposuction is more about fat than about skin. The more elastic your skin, the better result you will get. If you have flabby skin caused by pregnancies, ageing or weight fluctuation, liposuction can potentially leave you looking ripply.

The procedure

Tiny incisions (3–6 millimetres) are made and a wetting solution is infused to anaesthetise, reduce bleeding and improve fat extraction. The surgeon uses a cannula – a hollow, thin, tube-like instrument with holes at one end to trap the fat. The cannula is attached to suction tubing through which the fat is evacuated. It is inserted under the skin and moved back and forth in a criss-cross fashion within the fat, pushing it aside while protecting the vessels and nerves. The fat is suctioned out through the holes at the tip and measured. Your body is then checked for symmetry.

Time in operating theatre

Two to four hours.

Post-op effects and recovery time

Significant swelling immediately after the procedure subsides within a few days. You will weigh more right after lipo than before. Your face, feet and hands may swell up from the fluids pumped into you. Swelling travels downwards, so don't be surprised if you're puffy in places you didn't have suctioned; for example, you may be swollen around your knees if your inner thighs were sucked out. You will also have numbness and itching as nerve endings wake up. Using a rich moisturiser and a loofah in the shower and taking warm oatmeal baths can soothe dry skin. You will need to wear a girdle-like garment for several weeks. You can be up and about within a few days, and resume exercise pretty much as soon as you want. Wait at least six weeks before having clothes tailored or buying smaller sizes, as you will still be swollen. You will look better three months after lipo than you do at one month, as the remaining swelling settles.

GIRDLES

Specially designed stretch support garments are worn for two to six weeks after body contouring procedures (liposuction, tummy tucks, bodylifts). A properly fitted compression garment is an essential part of the recovery process. It can improve skin retraction, minimise swelling and keep you comfortable. Black is preferable to nude or white, since staining is hard to remove. Purchase at least one extra garment to switch to when you rinse the first one out (they cannot be put in the dryer). You may also need a smaller size when your body shrinks. See www.wear-with-all.com, www.surgical-garments.com, www.design-veronique.com.

Your Lovely Lower Half

145

Risks

Risks are usually related to the expertise of the surgeon and the anaesthetist. Specific risks include rare complications such as pulmonary edema, which is a collection of fluid in the lungs that may occur if too much fluid is given. A fat embolus can also occur where a bit of fat travels into the bloodstream. Another potential complication is lidocaine toxicity, when there is too much lidocaine in the solution. If too much solution is injected, overworking your heart and essentially drowning from too much fluid are possible consequences. Anti-embolism boots are often used during surgery to prevent a blood clot from forming in the deep veins of the pelvis or legs. The risk of a seroma, or collection of fluid, is more common in some areas, such as the tummy, and fluid may have to be drained to relieve pressure. If needed, a touch-up may be done six months after the initial procedure to take out a little more fat.

How long it lasts

Results are permanent, as long as you keep your weight stable. If you gain weight after liposuction, it will tend to show in the areas not suctioned, where fat cells will continue to expand.

Minimum spend

£4,000–8,000.

Optimum age

The younger, the better, while skin is still springy and can snap back nicely. It is possible at any age over 18.

Ouch factor

2.

What is the alternative?

Fat-dissolving injections and non-surgical fat reduction, as well as tummy tucks and bodylifts if there is excess skin or fatty deposits that need attending to.

Denise's near-death experience

Surely everyone in the UK has heard about the horrific liposuction that nearly killed a footballer's wife. Essentially, she went in for liposuction of her stomach after having four children, and her bowel and colon were punctured multiple times, causing blood poisoning and organ failure. She spent five weeks in a coma and nearly two months in intensive care, but fortunately lived to speak about it. Puncturing happens very rarely during liposuction and in this instance occurred because of a technical error made by the surgeon, who perforated her bowel by plunging a fat-sucking instrument too deeply. The moral of the story is that even a simple operation can become life-threatening when an incompetent doctor is at the helm, so choose your surgeon carefully.

QUICK-FIX LIPO

LipoSelection® By VASER

The procedure

You may already think that fat-sucking methods are a dream come true, but a physicist has now developed a technique that targets just your fat cells and leaves other structures intact. LipoSelection® by VASER utilises ultrasound technology to create a more precise way of separating fat from your body than traditional lipoplasty. Fat pockets are quickly dissolved and then safely swept away, and the possibility of uneven contouring, ripples, lumps and bumps is reduced. Recovery is faster, and the procedure minimises bruising and maximises smooth skin retraction, but it is still a surgical procedure.

Recovery time

You can usually return to normal activities after a long weekend.

Risks

Safety has been well established with this technology.

How long it lasts

Permanent if you keep your weight stable.

Costs

£3,000 and up, depending on how many areas are treated, not including hospital and anaesthetist.

Manufacturer

VASER®, US, www.vaser.com.

Smartlipo®

The procedure

Smartlipo® is a method of minimally invasive liposculpture treatment that utilises cannulae, which have a diameter of only one millimetre. The process is called Laserlipolisi®, and it is a less traumatic technique for removing localised fat deposits than traditional lipoplasty. The Nd:YAG laser device breaks up the membranes that surround your fat cells, pulverising them into an oily liquid that is absorbed and eliminated through your natural bodily systems. A general anaesthetic is not required, and it can be done in your doctor's consulting room.

Recovery time

Recovery is faster than with traditional lipoplasty, but smaller amounts of fat are removed. Most people can return to normal activities after a weekend.

Risks

Safety has been established with this technology.

How long it lasts

Permanent if you keep your weight stable.

Costs

£2,500 and up, depending on how many areas are treated in one stage.

Manufacturer

Dekalaser, Italy, www.dekalaser.com.

MELTDOWN: NON-SURGICAL FAT BUSTERS

Until recently the concept of getting rid of fatty bulges by injection has been just a flight of fancy but there are now several lipo alternatives being used and more under development that can literally vaporise your fatty globules with intense energy, not unlike industrial-strength vacuum cleaners. Developed to bypass the expense and recovery of lipo-suction, these devices deliver energy to destroy fat cells. The melted fat is eventually flushed away naturally or metabolised within about four weeks. Nothing invasive is required – no stitches, no scalpel – and there is no bruising and, best of all, zero pain. This works best for shrinking petite bulges rather than reducing you by a few jean sizes.

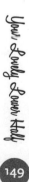

Your Lovely Lower Half

UltraShape™ is the first of these devices; the next ones coming are called Smooth Shapes® and Liposonix®, and there are more on the way.

UltraShape™ Contour 1 and 2

The procedure

UltraShape™ is a painless, non-invasive way to lose fatty tissue. Ultrasonic energy is applied directly to the skin's surface to disrupt and selectively reduce fatty tissue.

Recovery time

Literally no side effects – no lie!

Risks

The biggest risk is that you won't see enough improvement and will need more treatments, which gets expensive.

How long it lasts

The fat cells are vaporised, but they will come back if you eat your way through a buffet.

Costs

About £1,000 per treatment. Three treatments are recommended; more are optional.

Manufacturer

UltraShape™, Israel, www.ultrashape.com.

TUMMY TUCK

What it does

Abdominoplasty, or tummy tuck, removes skin and fat from the middle and lower tummy and tightens the abdominal wall muscles. If your fat pouch is below the navel, a less complex procedure called a mini-tummy tuck or partial abdominoplasty may do the job. Tummy tucks may be combined with liposuction of the hips, waist or thighs for an even better contour. If you are planning future pregnancies, you may be advised to wait, as the vertical muscles in the abdomen are fused during surgery and will tend to separate again during pregnancy.

The procedure

The most common technique involves an incision made across the lower abdomen, just above the pubic area. This incision can be angled so that it can be concealed. A second incision is usually made to free the navel from surrounding tissue. Your skin is separated from the abdominal wall all the way up to your ribs, and a flap of skin is lifted to reveal the vertical muscles in your belly. The muscles are pulled close together and stitched into their new position. The skin flap is then stretched down and a wad of excess skin is removed. A new opening is sometimes made to create a new tummy button in the right position. The incisions are closed with sutures and/or staples.

Time in operating theatre

Three to five hours.

Post-op effects and recovery time

You may stay in hospital for two to three days. When you go home, your dressings will be replaced with an elastic binder that you will wear for several weeks. Bed rest is mandatory, with legs bent at the hips to reduce the strain on your tender tummy area. You may be up and around in a few days, but should avoid straining for three or four weeks. At first you may not be able to stand up straight without feeling a tugging sensation, but you should start walking as soon as possible. Most women can return to work after two weeks; three is better if you can swing it. Bruising is minimal, but swelling may take several weeks to settle down. Your tummy will be numb, hard and lumpy for a few months. Surface stitches are removed in five to seven days, and deeper sutures, with ends that protrude through the skin, will come out after two to three weeks. Vigorous exercise should be avoided until you can do it comfortably, within four to six weeks. It will take up to a year before your scars flatten, soften and fade out.

Risks

Possible complications include poor healing, skin loss, infection, asymmetries and the need for a secondary procedure. Drains are usually placed at either end of the horizontal incision. A seroma (pocket of fluid) is more common after a tummy tuck, and may need to be drained to speed healing. You can reduce the risk of blood clots by moving around as soon as possible after surgery. You will have a permanent scar, which may extend from hip to hip. The scar can be designed to remove any old ones, such as that of a Caesarean. The scar may be thick, raised and irregular. Occasionally, there is a projection of bulging tissue called a dog ear, which can be easily corrected.

Plastic Makes Perfect

How long it lasts

Results are permanent, but the skin will loosen up over time.

Minimum spend

£5,000–8,000.

Optimum age

Post childbirth or following large weight loss.

Ouch factor

3.

What is the alternative?

If you are willing to settle for loose skin but less fullness around your mid-section, liposuction may be enough. If you just have a small pouch of loose skin after pregnancies, skin tightening might give you a subtle improvement.

> ### A washboard tummy For Hillary
> At 44, Hillary thought she would never be a mother. She had tried to get pregnant for five years and had two miscarriages. Then one fine day, she found herself in the fertility specialist's chair and learned she was carrying twins. Hillary was delighted, but as her belly expanded, she began to worry if she would ever squeeze into size 8 clothes again. After giving birth to gorgeous twin girls, she shrunk by taking up kickboxing, yet she hated the crinkly skin and stretch marks that remained under her tummy button. For the girls' first birthday, her husband Paul wanted to get her a special present for all she went through to bring the twins into the world. She told him that she wanted her stomach done. Like a good husband, Paul said she didn't need it, but if that was what she wanted, he would go along with it. Hillary went in for her tummy

Your Lovely Lower Half

tuck and it was a great success. She could wear a bikini and felt sexy again, which made Paul pretty happy too.

LOWER BODYLIFT

To address the unsightly sagging skin left after massive weight loss, cosmetic surgeons have designed elaborate upper and lower bodylifts that literally pull up excess skin folds, just as a tailor takes in a coat and trousers. These are usually staged events; everything from the tummy down may be lifted in one go, and everything from the waist up may be reserved for a second or third round.

Scars are strategically placed in the groin and continue around the waist in a belt-like fashion. Additional scars may be needed to firm up the thighs and knees. Upper-body incisions may wrap around the upper back like the band of a bra, and bingo wings can be reshaped from the armpit to the inner elbow. In time, scars fade considerably and are rarely seen even when the patient is in a swimming costume. You can literally lose the size of an entire person from pre-stomach surgery to post bodylifting. For surgeons who do bodylift procedures, the satisfaction they feel is akin to restoring a woman's breast after cancer: it is very rewarding indeed.

What it does

Bodylifts are reserved for after significant weight loss, where there are unsightly loose pouches of excess skin. If you look in the mirror naked, and pull up the saggy skin of your hips to stretch out your upper thighs and abdominal area, you can see what a lower bodylift can do. It transforms the way your body looks by addressing the thighs, buttocks, abdomen, waist and hips all in one stage. The added benefits are an overall improvement in dimpling and cellulite – and a little tightening in your private parts too.

The procedure

Bodylifts are not for the squeamish. The procedure is performed under general anaesthetic and may require two or more nights in hospital and lots of aftercare. For thighlifts, excess skin is lifted and removed through incisions made in the inner thigh and/or high upper outer thigh. Simultaneous lifting of the thighs and buttocks is done using incisions that follow a line like a high-cut bathing-suit line only a bit higher up on the hip. The surgeon lifts and removes the excess skin down to the muscle and removes the thick layer of fat beneath the skin. Drainage tubes may be placed at the site of the incision. The scars can usually be somewhat hidden in the natural skin creases.

Time in operating theatre

Four to seven hours.

Post-op effects and recovery time

The recovery from a bodylift procedure is very similar to that for a tummy tuck, although healing can take longer, since the incisions are wider. You should try to walk as soon as possible (with assistance) to reduce swelling and prevent blood clots from forming in your legs. For the first week, you should avoid bending or lifting. The sutures will be covered with adhesive steri-strips, tape and surgical gauze, and some oozing and bleeding is common. Changing position at least every 30 minutes and moving around carefully will limit stress on the incision lines. You will have several layers of stitches with a bodylift procedure. Some will be resorbed by the body and some may need to be removed. Deep sutures will be permanent. You will usually be able to shower after a few days with some help. Numbness in small areas on the thighs is possible but usually disappears gradually over several months. Some swelling may remain for six months and up to a year. You can resume aerobic exercise such as jogging or contact sports within six weeks.

Risks

The scarring is significant and the healing process varies. Fluid can collect beneath the skin (seroma, hematoma) and may need to be aspirated with a needle. Infection and wound-healing complications including skin loss may occur during the first two weeks. There are risks of blood clots, infection, asymmetries, skin loss, prolonged numbness and delayed healing. This is serious surgery and the risks are greater than with most other cosmetic procedures. It is more than a tummy tuck – the scars are at least twice as long.

How long it lasts

Permanent – you don't want to do this twice!

Minimum spend

£8,000–15,000.

Optimum age

As needed, following multiple pregnancies or massive weight loss.

Ouch factor

4.

What is the alternative?

Tummy tucks, thighlifts and liposuction all fall under the category of alternatives to a bodylift, but they address specific areas and do not deliver the same effect. A bodylift is a massive undertaking, so brace yourself. But if you have loose skin dangling from these areas, the results can be truly transformational.

A beautiful bod for Maureen

After losing nearly five stone, Maureen was a shadow of her former self. She had gone from a voluptuous size 18 to a shrinking size 10 in less than a year through hard work and perseverance. There was just one problem she hadn't counted on: rolls of skin hanging from her belly, thighs and arms. Maureen almost felt she looked better when she was fat. Now she was slim, but she still couldn't show her body with confidence. Her moment of truth came when she saw a programme on television about a woman just like her who had had reconstructive surgery. The interesting thing was that her partner of ten years was totally against it. He felt threatened by Maureen's weight loss and insecure about the fact that she would now be attractive to other men. But Maureen was determined and wasn't going to let anyone hold her back. She researched the surgeon she had seen on television, got on a plane to America and checked herself into his clinic to have a bodylift. When she returned to England three weeks later, her partner had moved out. Maureen quickly got over him when a new man came into her life. She met him at, of all places, her gym. He noticed her sweating up a storm on the StairMaster® and came over to introduce himself. She will never forget the first thing he said to her: 'You are without a doubt the sexiest woman here.' It may seem like a cheap pick-up line, but to Maureen it was pure magic. 'Imagine me,' says Maureen, 'the sexiest!'

THIGHLIFT

What it does

A thighlift improves the look, shape and size of your thighs by doing away with the dimples and sagging. If you have droopy skin on your inner thigh, a thighlift will tighten and smooth out this area. The procedure can be performed with liposuction, which targets the outer thigh, to create a smooth overall appearance for the leg. To redrape slack skin on the outer thighs or saddlebag area, a buttock lift or lower bodylift may be indicated.

The procedure

A thighlift usually requires a night in hospital and a general anaesthetic. The surgery begins with an incision in the groin area, near the hip. The incision is made and the surgeon separates the skin on your thigh from the fat and muscle below by pulling the flap of skin upwards. Excess skin is removed and remaining skin is stretched back in place. Small stitches are made and the area is covered with bandages.
A drainage tube may be inserted in your skin.

Time in operating theatre

Two to four hours.

Post-op effects and recovery time

Recovery takes about one to two weeks, and you should plan not to return to work for seven to ten days. You will have a scar from hip bone to hip bone.

Risks

Spreading or widening scars and long-term numbness are possible, plus irregularities and loss of lift.

How long it lasts

Permanent, although ageing and gravity tend to cause scars to shift and laxity to return.

Minimum spend

£4,000–6,000.

Plastic Makes Perfect

Optimum age

Intended for after massive weight loss or where there is loose skin in the thigh area, at any age.

Ouch factor

3.

What is the alternative?

Liposuction of the inner thighs can help, but not if your skin is slack and uneven, in which case it may make it look worse. Lifestyle is a big factor: if you live in Scotland and rarely expose your thighs, it may not be a priority, but if you have a home in Provence, you may be more motivated to have a thighlift.

BUTTOCK LIFT

What it does

The ideal gluteal crease, where your buttocks join your thighs, should not go past two-thirds of the way across the thigh. A great backside should have a cute little dimple at the top, where the upper curve of the buns meets the base of the spine, so that it can peek out in low-rise jeans. You have three main muscles in your butt: the gluteus maximus, gluteus medius and gluteus minimus. They work together to help you move your upper legs in all directions. Every time you take a step, run for the tube, squat or jump, your rear is working for you.

Lifting the buttock involves reshaping and restoring a nice contour to the region. Particularly after losing a stone or two, the procedure can be used to smooth out the lower body and remove loose skin. Tightening up the skin above the upper part of the buttocks will lift you higher. I always smile when I hear about the trend towards bigger

Your Lovely Lower Half

A NEW ERA IN BODY BEAUTIFICATION

Barbed sutures are tiny threads (see www.quillsrs.com) that have microscopic little fingers or bristles that, when implanted in the skin, are used to yank up sagging tissues. The hottest wave in non-surgical face-, neck- and browlifting is showing up in places you would least suspect to find sutures – such as the glutes! Of course, the threads are thicker and more are needed to lift a wobbly bottom than to pull up a little skin on the cheek. They are also being used to lift droopy breasts and nipples that point to the floor, upper arms, hanging bums and crêpey thighs. There is a modest lifting effect, but the technology is being used to improve long-term results and wound closure for reshaping areas that show more skin slackening.

buttocks sweeping the nation. In the history of my career, I can count on the fingers of one hand the number of women who have come to ask me about making their bottoms bigger. In New York, we want no butts at all. A larger bottom is a very cultural phenomenon, and clearly more coveted in Latin countries. If your buttock is flat and you want more projection, you are better served with an implant or fat injections than a buttock lift. Fat injections give the butt more projection, volume and prominence. But if your bottom is sagging and sinking, fat injections can make it heavier and weigh you down. Rounder, fuller, higher buttocks with curves to rival J-Lo can be yours with a bit of silicone.

The procedure

Under general anaesthetic, an ellipse of skin and fat is cut out from the upper part of the buttock at the junction with the lower back. This allows for a true elevation of the buttock tissues and a reshaping of the entire butt. In combination with a liposuction of the hips or thighs this procedure can result in a dramatic reshaping of the entire backside. If your tush is the size of Trafalgar Square, you can first have liposuction to reduce the overall size of it and then a skin lift if needed. If you are having implants, the surgeon places a pair of special anatomically designed, solid silicone implants within the gluteus maximus. You don't actually sit on the implant because it is placed higher than the bones on which you sit. If your sag is minimal, a 'butt wedge' excision might be indicated – excess tissue is excised at the crease, leaving you with a scar where your thong goes.

Time in operating theatre

Two to four hours.

Post-op effects and recovery time

A buttock lift is not a pleasant experience, and it will be hard to sit or lie down comfortably after surgery. Your bottom will be tight and swollen, and getting around will present challenges. With implants, your buttocks will appear very full and boxy at first, and the implants will sit high in the buttock. As the swelling goes down, it will settle. You can return to work within two to three weeks.

Risks

Risks may include scarring, infection, problems with wound healing, blood or fluid collection and loss of sensation. The scar can migrate and spread over time. If you have fat injections, you may need more of them over time to keep up the effect. If you opt for an implant, it can shift, get infected or extrude, and may need to be replaced. The implant can rotate, which could be embarrassing; other risks include infection, scar tissue hardening and numbness.

How long it lasts

Five to ten years, barring pregnancy or excessive weight gain; implants may have to be adjusted, removed or replaced as time goes on and sagging develops.

Minimum spend

£4,000–7,000.

Optimum age

As needed; typically done post childbirth or following massive weight loss; can be done when younger to improve buttock contour.

Ouch factor

3.

What is the alternative?

Fat injections will fill out the butt and lift the buttocks. Liposuction for the saddlebags and banana rolls (the roll of flab under the buttock crease) can make your butt look smaller.

VAGINAL REJUVENATION

Just when you thought your plate was full enough worrying about sun spots, wrinkles and your impending waddle, there appears a whole new category of beautifying treatments to think about: designer vaginas.

How a woman perceives the way she looks down there can have devastating effects on her love life. It can threaten her self-esteem, reduce sexual desire and excitement or cause incontinence and discomfort. Multiple childbirths and ageing cause vaginal muscles to loosen, tear and weaken. The diameter of the vagina gets bigger and there can be a loss of sensation. In other words, along with your face, your uterus could be falling too. If you have ever leaked accidentally when laughing, coughing or sneezing, this surgery can help as it can also correct incontinence that occurs when your pelvis slacks off. Intimate surgery has both a cosmetic and a functional component.

What it does

Unless you watch a lot of adult movies, you're probably not familiar with the names of your private parts. Labia majora are the thick, fleshy structures that are usually covered with pubic hair. Labia minora are two small pink folds located inside the labia majora. The mons pubis is the soft mound of fatty tissue that sits above your pubic bone and is usually covered with hair. The perineum is the area just outside and below the entrance to the vagina. All these areas can be rejuvenated, enhanced, tightened or reduced upon request.

The procedure

Vaginal reconstruction can take the form of vaginoplasty (vaginal rejuvenation and tightening) and labiaplasty (labia reduction and enhancement). Hymenoplasty (reconstruction of the hymen) can return the ruptured hymen to a state of virginity. Cosmetic labiaplasty involves surgically reshaping the labia or improving the appearance of asymmetrical or deflated labia. A laser can be used for labiaplasty and vaginoplasty, to enhance vaginal muscle tone, decrease the vaginal diameter and strengthen the opening otherwise known as the birth canal. All these procedures are done under general or local anaesthetic.

Time in operating theatre

One to three hours; laser procedures are faster than traditional methods.

Post-op effects and recovery time

You can return to work within about one week, depending on what was done. With many nerve endings in these delicate areas, post surgery you can expect to feel tender and sore. Sex is off the table for six weeks, so inform your partner in advance that he will have to take cold showers.

Risks

Bleeding, infection, scarring and loss of sensation are possible.

How long it lasts

Long lasting, although future pregnancies and ageing will make things go south again.

Minimum spend

£3,000–7,000.

Optimum age

Women who have had children or who want to tighten their vaginal muscles.

Ouch factor

3.

What is the alternative?

Kegel exercises for your pelvic muscles are not brilliant. Fat, hyaluronic acid and other thicker fillers can be used to plump up fallen labia and bulk up the tissue surrounding the urethra to improve continence. Liposuction of the mons pubis can reduce and smooth this area.

WEIGHT-LOSS SURGERY

Obesity is a worldwide epidemic. According to the World Health Organization, more than 1 billion people are overweight, and at least 300 million are obese. As waistlines expand, minimally invasive stomach-altering procedures are becoming safer and more successful through less invasive endoscopic techniques.

Plastic Makes Perfect

What it does

Bariatric or weight loss surgery is not exactly a cosmetic procedure. It works by reducing the size of your stomach and/or digestive tract to limit your intake of calories, causing you to shed the kilos. Currently, there are three main techniques available:

- Roux-en-Y gastric bypass
- Biliopancreatic diversion bypass
- Lap banding.

The biggest weight loss is often seen from gastric bypass operations that cause malabsorption and restrict food intake. Bypass operations can cause you to lose two-thirds of your weight within two years. Restrictive operations, which are more common, only decrease food intake.

The procedure

Bypass operations:

Roux-en-Y Gastric Bypass (RGB) The Roux-en-Y bypass is more common and less complicated than the biliopancreatic diversion bypass, since it does not remove portions of the stomach. It can be performed through open surgery with one long incision, and also laparoscopically using multiple smaller incisions, which lets you recover faster.

Biliopancreatic diversion bypass (extensive gastric bypass) This technique is done through open surgery with one long incision, leaving a permanent scar. It is less common, since portions of the stomach are removed and the bypass is attached to the intestine. This technique significantly restricts food intake and reduces hunger to promote healthy weight loss for the first one to two years.

Restrictive surgery:

Vertical gastric banding During the procedure, referred to as 'stomach stapling', both a band and staples are used to create a smaller stomach pouch.

Gastric banding A band is placed around the stomach near its upper end, creating a small pouch and a narrow passage into the larger remainder of the stomach so that you have to eat and drink less.

The LAP-BAND® system This adjustable system has three band sizes to fit different sizes of stomachs, and can be placed endoscopically, which makes it more appealing than more invasive methods.

Time in operating theatre

One to two hours.

Post-op effects and recovery time

After gastric bypass surgery, one to three days in hospital and two to five weeks of recovery are needed. Your abdomen will be swollen and sore. Aftercare typically includes a strict dietary plan, regular exercise, behavioural-modification therapy and vitamin supplements. After restrictive surgery, food intake is significantly limited and food has to be well chewed. Eating massive amounts of food at one time is a thing of the past; you will nibble on several (eight to ten) small meals throughout the day instead. This takes a little getting used to.

Risks

Risks include malnourishment and infections. Even with a reduced stomach, you can regain all the weight if you eat poorly and don't exercise, which occurs in about five per cent of cases.

How long it lasts

Weight loss continues for up to one to two years.

Minimum spend

£7,500 and up; in some cases gastric bypass and lap banding may be covered by private health insurance, if you can prove that other methods have failed and your health is at risk.

Optimum age

Adults are the best candidates, although weight loss surgery is done on teens in extreme cases of obesity.

Ouch factor

2–3, depending on the method selected.

What is the alternative?

The LapBand®, which is an adjustable stomach-restricting device, is thought to be safer than other methods. The Intragastric Balloon® system (see right) is considered an alternative to more invasive and long-term procedures.

THE SHAPE OF YOUR FUTURE

You've taken the plunge and had it all done. It probably wasn't exactly a day at the beach, but your body looks half its age and you want to flaunt it in Lycra and spandex. Now what can you do to keep up the results and hang on to your thinner thighs and bootylicious bum? Invest in a nutritionist to set a sensible programme to help you maintain your new shape. Join a gym near your work or home so that you can get there easily, and hire a trainer to help get you going and sort out your workouts so that you can get the most benefit from working up a sweat. Lipo-suction and bodylifts are not substitutes for healthy living. Any major weight gain and loss will stretch out the skin and cause it to sag sooner than expected.

Your Lovely Lower Half

Ask The Beauty Junkie®

Can you gain weight after liposuction?
Liposuction removes some but not all of your fat cells. If you gain weight after liposuction, you may gain weight in other areas as well. Liposuction is not a substitute for diet and exercise. Minor irregularities can be corrected or evened out as needed, but you may have to wait three to six months for any revisions.

Does liposuction get rid of cellulite?
Cellulite is not garden-variety fat. It lives deep within the septa, where liposuction cannulae typically cannot reach. Lipo can make your thighs, buttocks and hips look smoother, but it isn't a cure for cellulite.

What is the difference between a breastlift and a breast reduction?
The techniques are similar; however, usually with a breastlift the size of the lifted breast is the same or smaller than before surgery. In a breast reduction, more breast tissue (fat, glands) and excess skin are removed, to make the breast size smaller. A breast reduction also lifts the breast and creates a more youthful shape. Generally, a breastlift is a less involved procedure because less tissue is being altered. However, a breastlift can also be accompanied by the placement of an implant if needed.

What is a mini tummy tuck?
For resistant fat pockets on the abdominal wall, loose skin, and stretch marks on the lower abdomen, a mini tummy tuck may be an alternative to a full abdominoplasty. A mini tummy tuck may be done alone or can be paired with liposuction of the abdomen, hips or thighs to restore good contour and a trimmer waistline. The advantages of a mini tuck are that the scar is somewhat shorter vertically. It is ideally suited for smaller tummy bulges where there is not too much excess skin or fat.

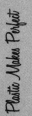
Plastic Makes Perfect

Can you have fat removed from your hips and put into your breasts?

Some doctors use your own fat to enhance the size and shape of your breasts. However, based on potential risks, this is quite a controversial procedure, Proponents of this concept ascribe to the theory that autologous tissue (your own) is best. Fat is being placed to add cleavage, enhance the upper area of fullness that gets lost with age and pregnancies, and to repair asymmetric or tuberous (irregularly shaped) breasts. There is research being done to consider the safety issues of injecting fat into reconstructed breasts to restore fullness.

Part III

THE TUCK WITHOUT THE NIP: COSMETIC SURGERY LITE

The advent of innovative non-surgical procedures that mimic the effects of surgery at reduced costs, and with reduced risks and recovery times has revolutionised the anti-ageing world. If the idea of no-knife facelifts with fillers, threads and skin-tightening machines appeals, there are many techniques on offer that do a lot more than the micro-current non-surgical facelifts that were once the gold standard in the UK.

Our never-ending pursuit of a natural result without the telltale signs of surgery has led to a whole new generation of minimally invasive devices and techniques. They can deliver results that won't elicit remarks like 'What did she have done?!' For some, these treatments can help to delay the recourse to the knife. The philosophy is to have smaller procedures at a younger age to put off the need for more drastic nips and tucks until later on. You can make small, subtle changes that allow you to stay on top of the ageing process, and save surgery for when your sagging is out of control.

CROSSING THE POND

Europe is light years ahead of America in terms of breast implants and fillers. These are classified as medical devices, and get approval much more easily in the EU than via the US FDA, which can take four years and as many millions. In Europe, the burden is on the manufacturer to demonstrate quality, safety and performance, but the standards are very general. This cavalier attitude stimulates innovation but also paves the way for unsafe products and technologies to creep into the market. America leads the way in lasers, light devices and cosmetic dentistry. However, in recent years, devices have crossed the pond much faster than they used to, so European doctors are able to purchase the newest lasers pretty soon after their American counterparts. US cosmeceutical brands are also cropping up in Harvey Nichols and Selfridges much quicker than they used to.

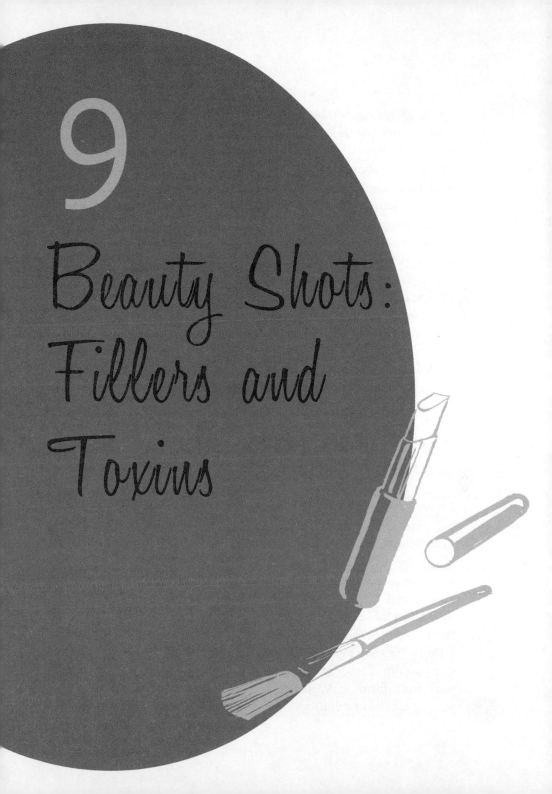

9

Beauty Shots: Fillers and Toxins

The global market for cosmetic fillers that plump up wrinkles and lines, rejuvenate faces, reshape chins, and create cheekbones and voluptuous lips has been estimated at almost £250 million. America accounts for about half of the market (and half of that is probably in New York, Los Angeles and Miami). It's no wonder that such a flurry of activity surrounds every new thing that can fit into a syringe. Beauty shots are big business indeed.

Fillers and Botox® – botulinum toxin – have become mainstays to reverse the signs of tired-looking faces. Their benefits no longer stop where the chin meets the neck. If it moves, you can have it immobilised; if it deflates, it can be filled up; and if it droops, you can lift it. Injectables can be artfully used to add volume to lift the mid-face and jawline, beautify features and camouflage flaws.

Immediate gratification is the hallmark of an injectable beauty procedure. It is truly amazing how plumping up wrinkles, creases and folds can instantly transform your look. It's a real confidence booster!

What is the difference between Botox® and fillers?

Every new filler that hits the market somehow gets tagged 'the new Botox®', yet Botox® is not a filler such as collagen or fat. It relaxes muscles to make lines disappear and can slow down the formation of new lines. Most fillers temporarily plump up creases but don't prevent them from getting deeper or stop new ones from forming. With fillers, your muscles are still fully active.

FILLERS VS. TOXINS

Fillers are considered medical devices in Europe; toxins are drugs. This sheds some light on why there are only three toxins on the market, and over 70 fillers. Getting approval for medical devices is much faster, cheaper and easier than meeting the requirements for bringing a new drug to market.

Fillers are used to add volume to the face, which Botox® cannot do. Fillers work better in deep creases and cheeks, and in the lips. These treatments are not mutually exclusive; they go hand in hand.

What is your filler filling?

Botox® is the hero among devotees for the brow area. This is also the area most commonly done. If the creases between your brows are very deep, fillers can come to the rescue, but a toxin is usually the first course of treatment. Since Botox® has taken over, fillers are used less frequently for the forehead and around the eyes. Botulinum toxin is not always as effective on lines that are not entirely caused by the action of a muscle. For example, the nasolabial folds (nose-to-mouth lines) are formed by muscle action and the weight of sagging skin. Some areas can't be treated because the muscles are needed for things like eating, kissing and opening the eyes. For deeper wrinkles, you may need a one-two punch toxin and filler combination. In general, static wrinkles are best treated by fillers and dynamic wrinkles by toxins.

Fillers and toxins are not just for wrinkles any more. They can also be used for a head-to-toe makeover. Some of the most innovative uses are still experimental, but could prove exciting.

- **Lift brows** – drooping eyebrows can be tweaked and asymmetric eye-lids can be subtly altered by Botox®; the brow bone can also be enhanced with fillers.
- **Smooth under-eye hollows** – Restylane® and fat can be injected into under-eye padding to give the area some volume and decrease dark circles.
- **Plump up thin earlobes** – saggy, deflated, old-looking earlobes drooping from wearing too much bling for too long can be filled in with Restylane® or HydraFill®.
- **Fill out flat cheeks** – Sculptra® and Restylane® SubQ can restore the curves and fullness of youthful cheeks.
- **Tip up long noses** – Botox® can be injected to raise the tip of a nose that is pointing towards the toes; fillers such as Radiesse® can fill out a small or pinched tip, dents and divets in the nose, to avoid having another op to fix a nose job gone wrong.

- **Reshape chins** – Restylane® and other fillers can round out a pointy chin or add volume to a receding one.
- **Improve smiles** – Botox® will help the muscles relax and hide gums when you smile.
- **Lift necks** – Botox® will relax some of the muscles under the chin to lift and reshape the area.
- **Smooth décolletés** – Botox® is injected directly into the body of the muscle to smooth out vertical creases.
- **Perk up mammaries** – Botox® may give breasts a perk by relaxing the pull of the pectoralis (chest) muscle and raising the nipples.
- **Perk up nipples** – ArteFill® and Radiesse® can perk up nipples that are pushed in.
- **Rejuvenate hands** – Botox® is being used to camouflage bulging veins and Restylane® Vital can improve skin texture.
- **Soften scars** – injecting scars with Botox® as they heal will soften and improve scars and minimise telltale signs of surgery.
- **Fend off food cravings** – Botox® can inhibit the nerve impulses that trigger your appetite.
- **Banish incontinence** – Botox® may be injected into the main muscle of the bladder to relieve incontinence.
- **Iron out cellulite** – Restylane® and HydraFill® can be injected to rid your legs and buttocks of pesky dimples.
- **Slim calves** – Botox® can help overused muscles relax.
- **Rejuvenate feet** – Restylane® Perlane or Sculptra® is injected into the soles and pressure points to help Jimmy Choos stay on with ease.
- **Lessen facial tics** – Bell's palsy, trauma and facial surgery mishaps can be lessened with Botox®.
- **Sensitise G spots** – injecting this highly sensitive area behind the pubic bone with a

> ## PRE-INJECTION TIPS
>
> - Avoid aspirin products (Nurofen, ibuprofen), blood thinners or vitamin E for one to two weeks before treatment to prevent increased bleeding and bruising.
> - Don't have a treatment on an empty stomach – you may get dizzy or faint.
> - Ice packs before and after help with pain and swelling.
> - Bring concealer with you to cover up bruises or needle marks.

filler is said to enhance female stimulation.

- **Bingo wings** – Sculptra® can be injected to firm up the sagginess of upper arms.
- **Taper jawlines** – Botox® injected into your massete muscles, the ones that help you chew, can taper the jawline or even stop you from clenching your jaw.

PAIN-FREE FILLING

NIP TIP
Ask your doctor for a caine-based product such as BetaCaine®, EMLA® 5 per cent, LMX4® or AneStop®. Apply it to the area to be injected prior to having your injection and leave it long enough for the skin to get numb. For lips, a dental block is a welcome addition to treatment. Highly recommended!

I am always aghast at the arguments I hear at medical conferences on the topic of pain management. Needles hurt – that point is rarely disputed. The thinner the needle, the less you feel the injection. You can get a long way with an ice cube, too, especially if it comes with a little Stoli. 'Talkesthesia', or vocal anaesthetic, sounds good on paper. It is equivalent to a man telling you to breathe deeply while the head of your 4.5 kg baby is passing through your birth canal. Why not exercise your right to have a filler session that does not leave you crying out in pain? There are many little steps you can take to maximise your comfort during an injection and keep you relaxed and comfortable. For starters, ice packs are heaven sent.

In the scheme of discomfort from fillers, lip augmentation is by far the worst. The Cupid's bow (the upside-down W-shaped bit in the centre of the top lip) and the corners of the mouth sting the most. Your doctor can inject the upper gums by the nasolabial folds with an anaesthetic to take the burn away from the injections. The added measure of a simple little dental block that takes a few seconds to do can make the difference between having your lips done every six months and never ever coming back. A variety of these nerve blocks can be used to anaesthetise the lips, around the mouth, the cheeks, nose and lower eyelids, and jawline. They provide temporary pain relief that makes them ideal before having fillers done.

Beauty Shots: Fillers and Toxins

177

How much toxin or filler do you need?

My general theory when it comes to toxins is that less is more. For the upper face (brows, forehead, eyes) you usually need a sizeable dose to get the full effect, but not so much that you are overdone. If you have too little, you may think your Botox® isn't working, which is rarely true. For the lower face (around the mouth, chin, neck) you need precious little. But when it comes to fillers, it is often a case of more is more. One syringe of collagen or hyaluronic acid won't go very far or last very long if you have a few sets of lines to treat. If you have really thin lips, two syringes is a must; ditto for deep nasolabial folds. In your thirties, you may get away with a syringe here and there. In your forties, two is the norm. In your fifties, the sky's the limit.

BOTULINUM TOXINS

No other single product has revolutionised cosmetic medicine in such a relatively short time. Botulinum toxin has become the corner-stone of an anti-ageing programme for the face, and is usually the best treatment to begin with. It is the world's leading non-surgical aesthetic procedure.

Over 50,000 vials of Botox® are used in the UK annually, and that number is climbing rapidly. It is widely accepted that this is just the tip of the iceberg: a steady influx of new customers for injectable beauty fixes is expected.

Although to many people Botox® is just a vanity drug, it is a power-ful medicine because of the way it affects muscles and nerve endings. There is evidence that it interferes with the nerve signals associated with pain. Doctors are studying its effects on a whole spectrum of conditions including cerebral palsy, head, neck and shoulder pain, overactive bladder and knee pain from arthritis. One interesting discov-ery is that injecting Botox® in finger and wrist muscles can help writer's cramp.

At the current time, several botulinum toxin type-A formulas are marketed around the world, and there are a few more on the way. The leader is Botox®/Vistabel® (Allergan). Dysport®/Reloxin® (Ipsen/Medicis) comes next. A newcomer is Xeomin® (Merz, Germany). Puretox® (Mentor) is currently undergoing clinical trials in the US. There are also some other lesser-known brands that are licensed in selected countries only, including CBTX-A® (Lanzhou Biological Products Institute, China), and Neuronox® (Medy-Tox, Inc., South Korea). Linurase® (Prollenium, Canada) is reported to be undergoing testing for regulatory approvals in Canada.

Have a small treatment, and go back if you want a little more.

The case of the bogus Botox®

In 2004, there was a well-publicised case in Florida of a dodgy clinic doctor (not board-certified) who injected himself and three patients with unlicensed botulinum toxin and ended up in hospital. The product he used was never intended for use in humans, and was not diluted properly, so the concentration was off the charts. This was an incident of the misuse of a product that greatly exceeded the recommended dosage, which not surprisingly, had disastrous consequences. It was not the Botox® Vistabel® marketed by Allergan.

Botox® Cosmetic™ or Vistabel®

Botox® was a billion-dollar drug as of 2006, right up there with Viagra® as the world's best known.

The procedure

Botulinum toxin is injected in highly diluted doses into muscles, causing them to relax, which in turn softens lines and creases. The most popular

BOTOX® FOR BEGINNERS

If you're a first timer, start small with areas that always work well, even in the hands of less experienced injectors:
- The 'II's'vertical creases between the eyebrows (glabella)
- Crow's feet
- Horizontal forehead lines

areas are creases between the brows, crow's feet, forehead lines, neck muscles, corners of the mouth and upper lip lines, and new uses are being discovered all the time. Smaller needles are used for toxins than for fillers, so discomfort is quite bearable. Topical numbing cream can be requested.

Recovery time

Botox® is truly a wash-and-wear treatment; bruising is rare. It takes two to seven days to get the full effect.

Risks

It is rare but possible to get an eyebrow or eyelid droop, which will resolve on its own within two to three weeks. Asymmetries are possible and easily adjusted.

How long it lasts

Three to four months before the effects gradually wear off and muscle activity returns to normal.

Costs

£250 and up per area treated.

Manufacturer

Allergan, US, www.botox-cosmetic.com, www.thenaturallook.uk.

FDA status

Botox® Cosmetic™ is approved for cosmetic

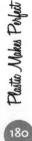

DON'T SWEAT IT

How do you think celebs stay so cool on the red carpet and under smouldering lights? Simple – it's Botox®! Excessive sweating (called hyperhidrosis) can be really embarrassing, not to mention expensive when you add up your dry cleaning bills. You may sweat profusely under your arms or have clammy palms and moist soles. When injected into the muscle, botulinum toxin reduces muscle tone, which alleviates the symptoms for six months or longer. It is an ideal alternative to painful, invasive surgical intervention.

use for glabellar/frown lines; other cosmetic uses are off label. Botox® is also approved for therapeutic uses.

EC status

Vistabel® received its licence in the UK for cosmetic use for glabellar/frown lines; Botox® is also licensed for therapeutic uses.

Dysport® or Reloxin®

The procedure

Several injections are made between the eyebrows or other facial areas to relax the facial muscles underlying the frown lines. No local anaesthetic is necessary but you may request numbing cream.

Beauty Shots: Fillers and Toxins

Recovery time

The procedure takes 15 minutes and requires no downtime.

Risks

Temporary soreness or mild bruising around the injection site; slight headache; small possibility of a drooping eyelid.

How long it lasts

Three to four months.

Costs

£250 and up per area per treatment.

Manufacturer

Ipsen Ltd, UK, www.ipsen.com; Medicis, US, www.medicis.com.

FDA status

Currently undergoing clinical trials in the US.

EC status

Licensed in the EU for therapeutic uses; cosmetic use is considered off licence, except in Germany and Russia, where it has cosmetic approval.

NIP TIP

If someone says, 'You look great – who does your Botox®?' you're busted! If your forehead looks 30 and your lower face looks 50, everyone in the know will just assume you've been Botoxed. Look at your whole face, and not just the parts that have the most lines and wrinkles. Overtreating one area while undertreating or ignoring another part of your face can make your face look unbalanced.

Puretox®

The procedure

Injected as other toxins into facial lines and wrinkles.

Recovery time

No downtime; possible bruise at injection site.

Risks

Uneven result, asymmetry, eyelid droop, tenderness, etc.

How long it lasts

To be determined, expect three to five months.

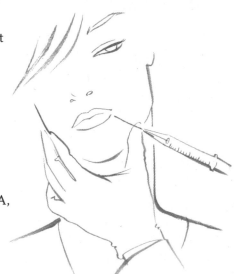

Costs

To be determined.

Manufacturer

Mentor Biologics, USA, www.mentorcorp.com.

FDA status

Currently undergoing clinical trials in the US.

EC status

None.

Beauty Shots: Fillers and Toxins

Xeomin®

The procedure

Xeomin contains no complex proteins, and does not require refrigeration. Because of this, it may be able to treat a small group of people who have not responded to other toxins.

Recovery time

No downtime.

Risks

Clinical safety profile suggests that it is comparable to other toxins on the market; studies are under way.

How long it lasts

Three to four months.

Costs

To be determined.

Manufacturer

Merz Pharma, Germany, www.xeomin.com.

FDA status

None.

EC status

Only approved in Germany for blepharospasm and cervical dystonia.

Alice's family furrow

Alice was starting to see two deep crevices forming between her brows. She blamed it on her constant squinting, since she didn't always wear her glasses for reading. Then she happened to notice in a family photograph that her older sister and her father were sporting the same nasty double crease. It turns out that facial expressions may be an inherited trait. A unique study from the University of Haifa in Israel found that the subjects studied showed similar facial expressions to those of their relatives. So perhaps that crooked smile, one arched brow or your signature scowl were inherited from your parents.

FILLERS

In Europe, there are more than 70 fillers on the market. I have listed only the safest and most popular fillers here, all of which have a CE mark (see page 243). Fillers with a high incidence of reactions and complications have difficulty getting approval from the US FDA. However, Europe and other parts of the world have less stringent criteria and fillers are often given approval based on limited clinical data.

Wrinkle fillers are a proactive way to address the early signs of ageing. But not all wrinkle fillers are created equal. There are two basic types of fillers: absorbable (temporary) and non-absorbable (permanent). The former are gradually broken down by the body while the latter are not. Temporary fillers include hyaluronic acids and collagens, both vital skin components that are lost as the skin ages. Longer-lasting temporary fillers include poly-L-lactic acid (Sculptra®) and fat. The most controversial varieties are the permanent fillers, such as injectable liquid silicone, and semi-permanent fillers, including hybrid fillers that contain teeny particles floating in hyaluronic acid or collagen. A general guideline is that the longer the filler lasts, the

NIP TIP
Be wary of any doctors who recap filler syringes – putting a new needle on a syringe that has already been used. Also make sure they wash their hands and wear clean gloves after the last patient leaves and you go into the room. Always insist that a new syringe is used for you; partially used syringes should not be saved for a top up at a later date.

Beauty Shots: Fillers and Toxins

greater the risks. Temporary, absorbable fillers that dissolve over time are widely considered to be the safest substances available.

There are some universal truths about fillers. All fillers can cause lumps, bruising and swelling – at least in some people some of the time. All the fillers on the market work to plump up lines and more. The big variables are safety, side-effects and how long they last.

THE HYALURONIC ACIDS

Hyaluronic acid is the new collagen. It is naturally found in the human body, so it is very biocompatible, and gets broken down over time. When injected into the skin, hyaluronic acid binds to water and adds sexy volume.

Restylane®

The procedure

The Restylane® family of hyaluronic acid fillers is growing: there is Restylane® Touch™ for fine lines, Restylane® for wrinkles, Restylane® Perlane™ for creases, Restylane® SubQ, which is implanted to build up chin and cheek contours, and the newest Restylane® Lipp™, which is just for lips. Each product is injected into a different layer of the skin, and products may be paired up for longer-lasting effects. Restylane®

FILLER FIASCOS

There is a possibility of side-effects from any filler:
- hardening and lumps
- chronic inflammation
- rashes
- extrusion
- migration
- infection
- allergic reaction
- acne

However, most are entirely avoidable and easily reversible or temporary.

celebrated its tenth birthday in 2006 and more than four million people have been treated worldwide. To find a qualified Restylane® practitioner, call 0800 015 5548.

Recovery time

Some swelling or bruising for a few days; make-up can be worn straight away.

Risks

Non-animal hyaluronic acid is naturally found in the body in the connective tissues and is safe and biocompatible.

How long it lasts

Six to nine months, depending on how much is used and what product is injected where.

Costs

£300 per syringe; two syringes are needed for multiple areas.

Manufacturer

Q-Med A.B., Sweden, www.restylane.com.

FDA status

Restylane® is approved for cosmetic use; Restylane® Touch (also called Fine Line) is pending FDA approval.

EC status

CE mark.

Restylane® Perlane

The procedure

Similar to Restylane®, Perlane is a thicker form of NASHA® gel which is injected into deeper wrinkles, lips and facial contours.

Recovery time

Instant results; some bruising is possible, as with all fillers.

Risks

Same as Restylane®; slightly thicker, so may produce more swelling.

How long it lasts

Six to nine months.

Costs

£300 and up per syringe.

Manufacturer

Q-Med A.B. Sweden, www.restylane.co.uk; Medicis, USA, www.restylaneusa.com.

FDA status

FDA approved.

EC status

CE mark.

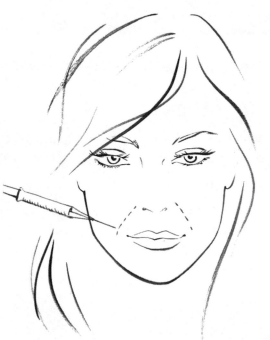

Restylane® SubQ

The procedure

Restylane® SubQ is a treatment for facial sculpting. It can produce the high cheekbones of a supermodel or a more defined chin and jawline without the need for hard synthetic implants that can shift and get infected. It has particles three times as thick as Restylane® Perlane™. The gel is implanted deeply under the skin under a local anaesthetic. SubQ can also be used for restoring facial volume where cheeks have hollowed from weight loss and suffered the inevitable breakdown of collagen and elastin fibres that plagues us all.

Recovery time

Mild bruising, redness and swelling are possible for a few days; results are immediate.

Risks

Non-animal hyaluronic acid is biodegradable, and the body breaks it down over time.

How long it lasts

8–12 months.

Costs

£600–1200, depending on the extent of the treatment.

Manufacturer

Q-Med Esthetics,
www.restylane.com.

FILLERS FOR BEGINNERS

Are you a filler virgin? A wide-eyed newbie? Then start small with areas that are easy to fill and have a high satisfaction rate:
- nasolabial folds
- oral commissures
- lip border

Have only one syringe to start with, and go back for a bit more in two to three weeks if you need it.

FDA status

Clinical studies are under way.

EC status

CE mark.

Macrolane®

The procedure

Macrolane® is approved to fill out indentations on the body and certain scars, such as asymmetries after liposuction. It is hyaluronic acid, the same substance that has been used to fill out wrinkles and enhance lips. Another Macrolane® product is also being investigated for shaping and enhancing breasts. This can be injected directly into the breast to give small to moderate enlargement of the breast without implants.

Recovery time

Results are immediate and you can resume normal activities. Avoid strenuous activity for a few weeks, including constant pressure in the treated area.

Risks

Swelling, tenderness, pain and bruising may occur. Typically these reactions resolve in one to two weeks; however, onset may be delayed and may last for longer.

How long it lasts

Up to 12 months after initial treatment.

Costs

Depends on the amount of product used.

Manufacturer

Q-Med AB, Sweden, www.q-med.com.

FDA status

None.

EC status

CE certification for concave body deformities.

Juvederm Ultra™

The procedure

The Juvederm Ultra™ Range combines smooth, 3D matrix technology with lidocaine to create a unique range of highly pure hyaluronic acid dermal fillers and skin rejuvenation products. This next generation smooth consistency gel delivers a natural look and feel that lasts. The lidocaine aids in the comfort of the injections, which is ideal for the needle phobic.

Recovery time

There may be swelling or bruising, but make-up can be worn straight away.

Risks

As this is a non-animal hyaluronic gel, it is safe and biocompatible.

How long it lasts

Up to 12 months.

Costs

£300 per ml syringe.

Manufacturer

Allergan, US, www.thenaturallook.co.uk

FDA status

FDA approved for cosmetic use.

CE status

CE mark.

> **ADVANCED FILLING**
>
> Veteran fill-ee? Feeling brave? Now see what other areas can be improved and recontoured with clever use of fillers. They can be used for:
> - filling in jawline 'parentheses'
> - cheekbone enhancement
> - nasal refinement

Elevess™

The procedure

Elevess™ is an injectable dermal filler used for the treatment of wrinkles, scars, and lip augmentation. It will contain an anaesthetic to reduce the discomfort of injections.

Recovery time

Some swelling for a few hours or days.

Risks

As with all hyaluronic acids, swelling, bruising, redness, pain and tenderness may occur.

How long it lasts

Approximately 6–12 months.

Costs

$300 per treatment.

Manufacturer

Anika Therapeutics, www.anika.com, Galderma, www.galderma.com

FDA status

FDA approved.

EC status

CE mark.

Puragen® and Puragen® Plus

The procedure

Whereas other hyaluronic fillers are made of single cross-linked molecules, Puragen® features double cross-linked hyaluronic acid molecules. This double cross-linked hyaluronic acid gel filler is supposed to last longer.

Recovery time

Some swelling for a few hours or days.

Risks

Some swelling, redness, pain, itching, discolouration or tenderness may occur at the injection site.

How long it lasts

Six months or longer, depending on how much is injected.

Costs

£300 per 1 ml syringe.

Manufacturer

Mentor Biopolymers/Genzyme Biosurgery, US, www.mentorcorp.com.

FDA status

Pending FDA approval.

EC status

CE mark.

WHAT TO KNOW BEFORE YOU USE A FILLER

- What is the source of the material?
- Is it natural, animal or synthetic?
- How long has it been on the market?
- How long has the doctor been using it?
- What is the name of the manufacturer and where are they located?
- What kinds of clinical studies have been done?
- What are the possible side-effects?
- Could I be allergic to it?
- What does a reaction look like and how long does it last?
- What can be done if I have a reaction?
- How many treatments will I need and how often?
- How much will each treatment cost?
- If it doesn't look right, what can be done?
- Can I still have other fillers later on?
- Is it FDA-approved?
- Is the manufacturer planning to apply for FDA approval in the near future?
- Is it licensed for cosmetic use?

Prevelle®

The procedure

Non-animal sourced hyaluronic acid gel filler injected for fine lines.

Recovery time

Instant effects, no downtime.

Risks

Minimal risk of swelling, redness, pain, itching, etc.

How long it lasts

Three to six months, depending on how much is injected.

Costs

£200 per 1 ml syringe.

Manufacturer

Mentor Biopolymers/Genzyme Biosurgery, US, www.mentorcorp.com.

FDA status

Pending FDA approval.

EC status

CE mark.

Beauty Shots: Fillers and Toxins

Teosyal®

The procedure

This Swiss gel range comes in several formulas of varying thickness, the different thicknesses dictating where they go and what they are used to plump and fill.

Recovery time

Possible swelling or bruising; make-up can be worn straight away.

Risks

Temporary discomfort including redness is possible.

How long it lasts

Six to nine months, depending on how much is used.

Costs

£250–400 per treatment.

Manufacturer

Teoxane Laboratoires, Switzerland, www.teoxane.com.

FDA status

None.

EC status

CE Mark.

Plastic Makes Perfect

Belotero®

The procedure

A monophasic, double cross-linked hyaluronic acid gel filler developed for lines, wrinkles, creases and scarring. There are two versions: Belotero® Basic for medium and deeper wrinkles and Belotero® Soft for superficial lines.

Recovery time

Instant results.

Risks

Hyaluronic acid gel fillers are safe for all skin types; some bruising and swelling is normal.

How long it lasts

Six months.

Costs

£300 per treatment.

> **LOSE THE LINES WITHOUT THE PAIN**
>
> Juvederm™ Ultra and Elevess™ will be the first hyaluronic acid gel fillers to include lidocaine for pain relief right in the syringe! Puragen® Plus is also on the table for the future. It looks like this will be the new trend.

Manufacturer

Anteis, Switzerland, www.esthelis.com; Merz, www.merz.com.

FDA status

None.

EC status

CE mark.

Collagen can come from farm animals, such as cows and pigs, as well as from humans and tissue banks. Since collagen is one of the main ingredients of the connective tissue layer, it seems logical to use it to fill up wrinkles in human skin.

Evolence™ and Evolence™ Breeze

The procedure

This long-lasting filler is made from pig's collagen. It is fortified with a natural sugar substance to increase its longevity, which involves a natural cross-linking process. This biodegradable filler is injected like other collagens, superficially into shallow lines and wrinkles. It can be used for wrinkles, lines, scars and lips, but may last 12 months based on the patented process.

Recovery time

There may be some mild swelling or bruising; since the injections are more superficial than some other substances, there is little downtime.

Risks

As this is an animal-derived product, there is a small risk of allergic reaction, but pre-testing is not required. If you have sensitivity to any other collagen product, check with your doctor before having it.

How long it lasts

Up to 12 months or longer, depending on how much is injected.

Costs

£300 per 1 ml syringe. A typical treatment is two syringes.

Manufacturer

ColBar LifeScience Ltd., Israel, a Johnson & Johnson company; www.evolence.com.

FDA status

Currently undergoing clinical trials in America for FDA approval.

EC status

CE mark.

Zyderm® and Zyplast®

The procedure

Bovine (cow collagen) is the mother of all fillers. Although many fillers have come and gone since the introduction of Zyderm® in 1982, it still has its diehard fans who will never switch. Zyderm® and Zyplast® collagens contain an anaesthetic, and are injected into lines and wrinkles.

Recovery time

Some swelling for 24 hours; make-up can be worn at once.

Risks

As this is a cow collagen product, a series of one or two allergy tests is recommended, spaced 30 days apart. Only three per cent of people are allergic.

How long it lasts

Three months.

Costs

£250 per 1 syringe. One or two syringes are needed.

Manufacturer

Allergan, US, www.allergan.com.

FDA status

Approved for cosmetic uses.

EC status

CE mark.

CosmoDerm® and CosmoPlast®

The procedure

These collagens use human collagen, which comes from cultured skin cells. They also contain lidocaine as an anaesthetic, which is a welcome addition if you're squeamish about needles. Unlike the fillers derived from cows, no allergy testing is required because the collagen is from a human source. CosmoDerm® works nicely to define the borders of the lips, for fine lines around the mouth and for smoker's lines.

Recovery time

Slight swelling or bruising; make-up can be worn straight away.

Risks

Excellent safety record; no skin test is needed, since it is human derived.

How long it lasts

Three to four months or longer, depending on how much is used.

Costs

£300 per 1 ml syringe. A typical treatment is two syringes.

Manufacturer

Allergan, US, www.allergan.com.

FDA status

Approved for cosmetic use.

EC status

Currently only available in certain EU countries including Germany, Italy, Spain and Switzerland as well as Israel, Australia and Canada, and some countries in South America and Asia.

FUTURE FIBROBLASTS

VAVELTA® is a new concept in facial rejuvenation products. It is a solution containing many millions of human dermal fibroblasts that comes in vials, which get injected into the skin to produce new collagen and improve imperfections. VAVELTA® is injected directly into the target area of the face using a fine gauge needle, requiring up to two one-hour sessions given four to six weeks apart. Currently undergoing clinical study, but coming soon to the UK from the cell therapy company, Intercytech Group. www.vavelta.com

Vicky's sunken cheek challenge

At 45, Vicky lost three stone through hard work and perseverance. The end result was a smaller tummy and waist, but her cheeks also seemed to deflate. Having had a pleasantly plump face for most of her life, she now looked gaunt and unwell. When I saw her she was considering cheek implants to give her face more roundness. Instead of hard implants that can slip or look unnatural and would require her to go to hospital, I recommended three treatments with Sculptra® to fill out Vicky's cheeks and hollows. One of the benefits of Sculptra® is that it stimulates new collagen growth and is a gradual process, so the effects appear over several months. We found her a good doctor near her home, and she was very pleased indeed in the end. I saw her again over a year later, when she was complaining about her lips deflating and looking older than her nicely contoured cheeks. I suggested Evolence® Breeze to enhance the shape of her lips and give her back a pretty pout. And the final touch was semi-permanent make-up to restore a natural looking rosy colour to her lips. Vicky's makeover was subtle and non-surgical and not even her children knew she had had an injection.

THE POLYMERS

Polymers are a new category of fillers, coming on the heels of the hyaluronic acids and collagens that preceded them.

Laresse™

The procedure

Laresse™ is a temporary filler made from pure, absorbable medical polymers. It is free of animal and bacterial proteins and is not cross linked, so it is biocompatible. Because there are no particles in the gel, only one formula is needed in superficial and mid-dermal layers; it is a

Plastic Makes Perfect

sort of one-size-fits-all filler. It is popular for lips and lip lines, and there is minimal swelling. It is a temporary filler and the gel is slowly absorbed over several months.

Recovery time

Some mild swelling or bruising; improvement is instant with little to no downtime.

Risks

As with any filler, temporary lumps are possible.

How long it lasts

Up to six months.

Costs

£300 per 1 ml syringe.

Manufacturer

Fziomed, US, www.laresse.com.

FDA status

Clinical studies under way.

EC status

CE mark.

Sculptra® (New-Fill™)

Sculptra® is a unique product. It is not a wrinkle-filler per se; rather, it is a volumiser, and it is considered a substitute for fat injections in some cases.

The procedure

Sculptra® is crystallised poly-L-lactic acid, a material that has long been used in dissolvable stitches. It is injected primarily to add volume to depressed areas such as creases, wrinkles, folds, pitted scars and sunken hollows around the eye sockets, temples and the mouth, and to plump up concave cheek areas. It is reconstituted with salt water and left for a few hours before use. Local anaesthetic can be added to ease the sting of the injection. The solution is shaken, not stirred, before it is implanted deeply into creases. Sculptra® works by increasing skin thickness by stimulating the body to produce new collagen. It has also been used on coarse wrinkles in the décolleté and to fill up ageing hands. A series of at least three treatments is needed for full correction. Treatments are done in one to two vials at one session, depending on how many areas are treated.

Recovery time

Some swelling and redness for 24 hours.

Risks

Lumps and bumps may occur if Sculptra® is injected too superficially; it is not an instant gratification product as it takes some time to see results.

How long it lasts

After three treatments, 18–36 months.

Costs

£350 and up per treatment.

Manufacturer

Sanofi-Aventis, France, www.sculptra.co.uk.

FDA status

Approved for HIV-related lipoatrophy; cosmetic approval is pending.

EC status

CE mark.

Radiesse®

The procedure

Radiesse® is composed of calcium hydroxylapatite, which is made up of calcium and phosphate. It is the same mineral component found in bones and teeth, so it is very biocompatible. Over time the tiny microspheres gradually break down and are absorbed into the body. Radiesse® is injected into the deep dermis to smooth out nasolabial creases, marionette lines, depressed scars and the chin area. It also works well for cheek enhancement, and to fill in scars and subtle nasal defects.

Recovery time

Some swelling or bruising; make-up can be worn straight away.

Risks

Mild irritation, edema, swelling, itching, discolouration or tenderness at the injection site may occur; not recommended for lips.

How long it lasts

Twelve months, depending on how much is injected.

Costs

£400 per 1 ml syringe.

Manufacturer

Bioform Medical, US, www.radiesse.com.

FDA status

FDA approved.

EC status

CE mark for plastic/reconstructive surgery, including soft tissue augmentation of facial area.

The Ultimate Filler: Fat

The procedure

Fat is extracted by syringe from your hips, tummy, thighs or wherever you have some, and then cleansed and re-injected into facial folds and creases, lips or hollows. This is a two-stage procedure: fat is harvested, then injected. Fat is ideal for larger-volume areas, such as the cheeks, chin, hollows, and areas that need to be built up. The treatment can be done in conjunction with facial surgery, or as a stand-alone procedure.

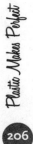

Recovery time

Swelling and redness for several days; bruising is likely since there is more trauma with fat transfer than with commercially available fillers.

Risks

Lumps and bumps may occur, as well as swelling, overcorrection, infection and asymmetries. If you are not happy with the results, it is hard to take fat out.

How long it lasts

Variable, from six months to several years, depending on the extent of the treatment; some doctors use large volumes of fat and inject it deeply into muscle tissue, which can be long-lasting and even permanent.

Costs

£1,500–5,000, depending on the extent of the treatment.

Manufacturer

Chips, crisps and Oreos®.

FDA status

Not required.

EC status

Not required.

NIP TIP
Avoid doctor hopping. When you find a good injector, stick with him. If you have several sessions of injections done by different doctors – each of whom has his own taste in beauty – you could start to look like a Picasso portrait.

Doctors talk of 'needle fatigue' among women whose faces are beginning to feel like pin cushions. For such women, a permanent filler may seem like a good idea. However, in the United States, doctors have never been great fans of permanent fillers. They are widely considered to be more tricky to use and more risky than their short-term cousins, and Americans' tolerance for risks and complications is nearly non-existent. If we feel even the hint of a lump we run back to the doctor or clinic to get it sorted.

'Permanent filler' is a misnomer. The only thing that is permanent about fillers is that they will remain in your body, whether you like it or not, until you are six feet under. Therein lies the critical difference: permanent fillers can produce permanent problems. Your face will continue to age around the permanent filler, so the effect is not really permanent.

NIP TIP

Women of a certain age have most likely tried several fillers over the years. Keep records of everything you have had injected and where – it is easy to forget. As a rule, permanent fillers should not be used where another permanent filler has been before. Come clean to your doctor about what you have had done to avoid any problems.

Artefill®

The procedure

The first permanent filler that has been granted FDA approval is ArteFill®. ArteFill® contains microscopic particles of something called polymethylmethacrylate microspheres (PMMA), which is a synthetic material similar to acrylic. The particles are suspended in cow collagen, arguably from a special, privileged herd of pampered cows. PMMA is not new: it has been used in dentistry and orthopaedics. The collagen is degraded by the body within about three months but the microspheres are left behind permanently. ArteFill® is implanted into the deep layers of the skin with a needle and then massaged and moulded to achieve the desired contour. It is used for acne scars, nasolabial folds, lips and building up cheek and chin contours. Previous generations of this technology were marketed as ArteColl® in Europe and Canada, but ArteFill® is a new formulation.

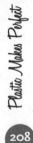

Plastic Makes Perfect

Recovery time

Results are instant; some swelling is to be expected.

Risks

There have been problems reported in the past of hardening and scar tissue formation.

How long it lasts

The collagen dissolves over three to four months, but the particles will remain permanently.

Costs

£500 and up per treatment.

Manufacturer

Artes Medical, US, www.artesmedical.com. ArteColl® is available outside the USA, and is made by Rofil, www.rofil.com.

FDA status

ArteFill® is approved for cosmetic use.

EC status

CE mark.

Aquamid®

The procedure

Aquamid® Injectable Implants are made from a polyacrylamide hydrogel composed of 97.5 per cent sterile water bound to 2.5 per cent

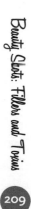

cross-linked polymers. They come in two varieties: Aquamid® for small lines and depressions, and Aquamid® Reconstruction for deeper lines, cheek and chin contours.

Recovery time

Avoid touching the treated area for at least six hours, and do not use cosmetics on the area for 24 hours. Avoid extreme heat and cold and prolonged direct sunlight for four weeks.

Risks

There is a risk of lumps, infection and migration. Bruising, tenderness and swelling are also possible.

How long it lasts

Long-lasting or permanent.

Costs

£400 and up per treatment.

Manufacturer

Contura International A/S, Denmark, www.aquamid.com.

FDA status

None yet.

EC status

CE mark.

Bio-Alcamid®

The procedure

Bio-Alcamid® is marketed as an injectable facial implant. It is a gel comprised of 96 per cent water and four per cent synthetic reticulate polymer, called a polyacrylamide. Immediately after the introduction of Bio-Alcamid®, a capsule is formed that encloses the substance so that it forms an implant. It is massaged into place.

Recovery time

Do not apply any pressure to the face for about a week, and avoid exposure to direct heat such as sunlight or hot water. Redness and temporary discomfort is to be expected, and more significant swelling and bruising.

Risks

Lumps, bumps and asymmetries are possible, and it may be tricky to remove if you are not happy with the results. There is a risk of potential migration of the substance under the skin.

How long it lasts

Results are long-lasting, but no specific duration is offered by the company.

Costs

£500 and up per treatment.

Manufacturer

Polymekon, Italy, www.bioalcamid.com.

FDA status

None.

EC status

CE mark.

Bioinblue™

The procedure

Bioinblue™ is a synthetic hydrogel consisting of six per cent polyvinyl alcohol (called PVA) and 94 per cent non-pirogenic water. It is supposed to be a soft consistency based on high water content, and is often used in the lips.

Recovery time

Do not apply any pressure to the face for about a week, and avoid exposure to direct heat such as sunlight or hot water.

Risks

Temporary discomfort including redness, swelling and bruising, and possible infection.

How long it lasts

Biodegradable, but long-lasting.

Costs

£300 per treatment.

Manufacturer

Polymekon, Italy, www.bioinblue.com.

FDA status

None.

EC status

CE mark.

Injectable liquid silicone

Silicone is a permanent filler that has been used since the 1940s. However, it was misused, and excessive volumes and non-medical-grade forms have caused complications and years of controversy among doctors. Medical-grade liquid injectable silicones are approved by the FDA for use in retinal detachments, thereby making silicone an off-label use for cosmetic purposes. Liquid silicone droplets are making a comeback. Silicone lasts forever, which has both

---

FILLER FIXERS

What can you do when a filler goes wrong?

Hyaluronidase An enzyme used to dissolve hyaluronic acid fillers; so if you get a lump you want to get rid of quickly instead of waiting for it to go on its own, your doctor can inject a tiny amount to settle it fast.

Corticosteroid injections Reserved for serious hardening and scar tissue, corticosteroids such as Kenalog® or 5 FU can be carefully injected to break up nodules.

Antibiotics If you are red and inflamed, you may have an infection where the filler was injected. See your doctor, who may recommend a topical or oral antibiotic such as a tetracycline.

Imiquimod Cream 5 per cent Also called Aldara™, this prescription-strength cream is used topically to treat granulomas.

pros and cons. Think of it like an oyster: there is a piece of sand in the shell and a pearl develops around it. The same thing happens with silicone: the little piece of sand becomes a fibroblast that starts to produce collagen to ward off this foreign substance. However, this reaction can cause lumps and scar tissue.

The procedure

Silicone is a man-made liquid that has been used in varying degrees of purity to treat wrinkles and scars for decades. Tiny injections called microdroplets are injected with small needles. The goal is to undercorrect initially, using small-volume injections, and similarly at each subsequent treatment session, at one- to three-month intervals, until the desired result is obtained.

Recovery time

Results are instant.

Risks

Once injected, liquid silicone is permanent. It cannot be removed easily, and in some cases, it cannot be removed at all. Silicone can create problems if too much is injected. Larger volumes can migrate with time, and because of the inflammatory reaction, bits of silicone will be difficult or impossible to remove. Less is definitely more.

How long it lasts

Permanent!

Costs

Varies.

Manufacturer

Silskin™, Richard James Inc., US, www.richard-james.com; Silikon 1000®, Alcon Labs, US, www.silikon1000.com; Adatosil 5000®, Chiron Corp., US, www.chiron.com; Surgisil™, US, www.surgisil.com.

FDA status

Approved only for retinal use; off-label cosmetic uses.

EC status

Not licensed in most EC countries; Permalip™ is CE marked.

READ MY LIPS

Lip augmentation is not just for women who want larger, sexier lips. As we age, our lips lose their fullness, which makes them appear older. Lip skin is very thin; it has three to five layers compared to facial skin, which has up to 16 layers. Lips have no oil glands, which accounts for why they dry out and chap. Lips descend because of loss of support. The distance between the tip of the nose and the upper lip gets longer.

The dreaded 'trout pout' look is not an inevitable consequence of having your lips enhanced. A great lip augmentation and rejuvenation addresses all of the following areas: the visible portion of the lip (the vermilion), the outer mouth (laugh lines), the edges of the lips (lipstick lines) and the inner lip. While most injectable fillers can tackle

LIP ANATOMY

- Vermillion – border between the lips and the surrounding skin
- Mucosa – mucous membranes that line the lips
- Philtrum – vertical groove on the upper lip
- Commissures – corners of the mouth
- Cupid's bow – double curve of the upper lip

this, some are more appropriate than others for each area. Temporary fillers are best around the mouth and along the border, and to redefine the edge and fill in lipstick and laugh lines. When fillers are injected into the inner lip, there is a greater chance of visible lumps and clumping. While injectable fillers combat ageing around the lips and mouth, some can lead to long-lasting problems if you're not careful.

Long-lasting fillers may remain for several years or permanently, and can leave you with overfilled lips that look obviously injected. Some fillers carry a higher risk of complications, which can result in the reverse effect of what you were hoping for. When you think of lip augmentation, you may immediately picture lips like Angelina Jolie's, but most people actually just need a subtle enhancement that adds curves and restores the lip border.

LIP TRICKS

Semi-permanent make-up, like a tattoo for your lips, can make thin, straight lips look fuller and more defined. Combined with volumising fillers, a touch of natural-looking pigment adds colour and shape to the lips. Lipstick and/or gloss can be used on top of semi-permanent pigment. It lasts a few years and can be topped up as needed. The colour looks darker at first, and then lightens up. Choose your technician carefully, by personal recommendation only, to avoid looking like Marilyn Manson.

Megan puckers up

After having thin lips like a boy's through her twenties, and never wearing lipstick, Megan longed to have a full, sexy pucker. Terrified of having lips like sausages, she went very lightly her first time. She had one syringe of what she was told was hyaluronic acid, but she didn't even know the brand name, and just had her upper lip injected. A few weeks later, her lip deflated. When she came to see me, she complained that it hadn't worked, and asked about something more permanent. The problem was obvious — she had been given an inferior product by an inexperienced injector and, of course, the results were disappointing. I referred her to a qualified practitioner and she had two syringes of Restylane® Lipp™ on her

Plastic Makes Perfect

top and bottom lip, which gave her pretty curves and a soft fullness. Megan was delighted. 'My boyfriend can't believe the difference it made, and it looks so natural.' She was so excited that she went to Space NK and bought herself a whole collection of lipsticks and glosses.

Lip plumpers

Restylane® Lipp™ is one of a new generation of specialised lip fillers. It is a soft, pliable and plumping hyaluronic acid that is specially designed just for lips. The advantages are that it is really soft and leaves the lips sultry and spongy, without hard lumps. It also is said to last longer – about six to nine months – so you can extend the time intervals between needles. Other specialised lip fillers on the market include Surgilips® and Teosyal® Kiss, which are temporary, and Permalip™, which is permanent.

FILLER FIASCO SOLUTIONS

- **Asymmetries** Go back for a top-up to even you out.
- **Lumps and bumps** With temporary fillers, massage and wait it out; with permanent fillers, say your prayers.
- **Gone before your cheque clears** Switch to a longer-lasting, thicker body filler or have more syringes.
- **Hurts like hell** Ask for a numbing cream or injection of local anaesthetic, apply ice and take two Panadol.

COSMETIC LIP FIXES

Not ready to go for a needle? Try these quick fixes to youthify your lips.
SkinMedica TNS® Lip Plumper – a two-step programme that nourishes and plumps with antioxidants www.skinbrands.co.uk
Freeze 2/47 Lip Plump – a cult favourite for plumping skinny lips in America and London www.freeze247.com

Ask The Beauty Junkie®

There are so many wrinkle fillers available, but how do I know which are safe?

The best-sellers in the filler world are hyaluronic acid gels. They are safe, give instant results and last around six months. Using your own fat is also popular, but recovery is longer and results are variable. More permanent fillers are more risky. Stick with products that have a good safety record and have been on the market for several years, not just a few months. Never be a guinea pig for the newest filler on the block.

How can I find a qualified Botox® injector?

In support of the Healthcare Commission's anticipated regulation of all clinics offering aesthetic procedures, in May 2006, Allergan launched a programme that offers practitioners who are existing Botox®/Vistabel® injectors the opportunity to come forward voluntarily to be validated for competency. As part of this programme, only injectors who successfully complete the voluntary Validation Programme will be presented with a UK Validation Certificate to be displayed in their clinics that attests to their competency to inject Vistabel®. Refer to Resources in the back of the book.

Do facial exercises really work?

Your face is the most exercised part of your body. It has 44 muscles and gets plenty of exercise every time your muscles contract and relax. Since these muscles are attached to the skin (as opposed to the bones or tendons, as other muscles in the body are) every time they move – when you speak, eat, laugh or cry – your skin moves. When you contract those muscles, the repetitive motion causes wrinkles. At the risk of going against tradition, in my humble opinion, exercising those muscles more will just accentuate your wrinkles. Over time, creases form where the skin contracted. The more you make the same facial movements, the deeper your lines get. The most compelling argument is that if facial exercises work, Botox® would not. Botox® stops muscles

Plastic Makes Perfect

from moving, which we know reduces lines, creases and wrinkles
– just look at my forehead on any given day for proof!

Is there surgery to enlarge lips permanently?

A lip lift can be done through an incision at the base of the nose
(called the columella) to lift the upper lip slightly so that the distance between the nose and top lip becomes shorter and the
upper lip appears fuller. There is another op called a cheiloplasty,
which involves making a scar along the upper lip line. It is not
commonly done because the scar is very noticeable and permanent and it can make your face look as though it has been through
a windscreen. Fillers are the safest and most predictable way to get
great lips.

Is Botox® addictive?

Botox® is like crisps – you can't have just one, because it is that
good. But to say that Botox® is addictive is like saying that lipstick
is addictive. If you have a Botox® treatment, it works, you like it,
and you go back for more – that is not a sign of addiction. An
addiction is classified as something that you need more of to
satisfy you with time. For example, if it takes two drinks to get a
sufficient buzz, you will need four drinks, and eight drinks, and
so on, to get the same buzz as you get addicted to alcohol. With
Botox®, the reverse is true. You need less as you go on because
there is evidence that muscles experience some long-term relax-
ation. So, you may start out having treatment every three to four
months, and later on your treatments may last four to five months,
so you may need less.

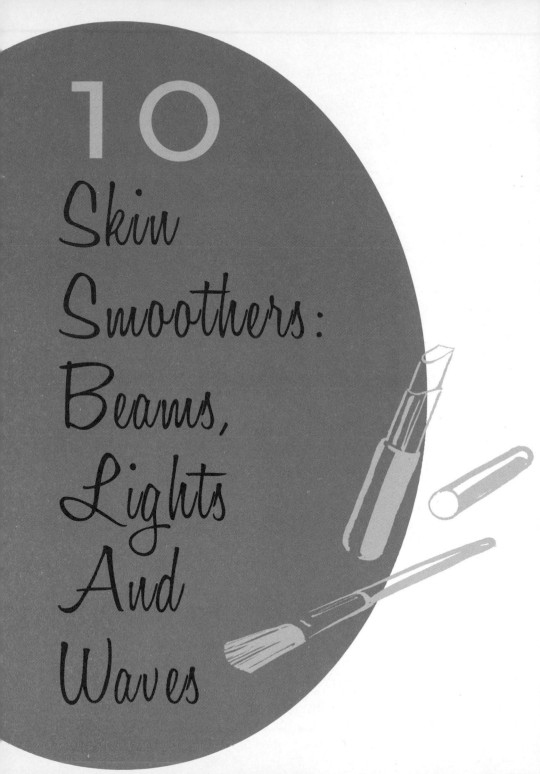

10

Skin Smoothers: Beams, Lights And Waves

Afraid of going under the knife? Terrified of being put to sleep? Nervous about going into hospital? The newest generation of devices includes Bond-like boxes with bells and whistles that can pulverise your wrinkles and age spots with the precision of a Scud missile.

SKIN RESURFACING

Resurfacing the skin can produce a whole myriad of improvements. These treatments are preventative as well as corrective.

Peels

The procedure

A chemical solution is applied to cleansed skin, left on for a period of seconds to minutes and then neutralised. The most common peeling agents are glycolic acid, beta hydroxy acid and trichloracetic acid (TCA).

Recovery time

Light peels may cause pinkness and mild flaking; deeper peels may result in peeling or crusting.

Risks

Side-effects may include skin lightening, skin darkening, blotches, scabbing, scarring, redness and blistering. The lighter the peel, the fewer the side effects.

How long it lasts

Superficial peels with glycolic acid are done in a course of treatments spaced three to four weeks apart; medium and deeper peels may be a one-off event.

Costs

£100–750, depending on the type of peel used.

Microdermabrasion

The procedure

A vacuum suction machine removes surface dead skin cells and exfoliates deeper layers of the skin to restore smoothness instantly – the wow factor is amazing!

Recovery time

No down time; slight pink colour like an afterglow.

Risks

Stinging and irritation are possible on sensitive skin.

How long it lasts

Results are temporary, and this is not a one-shot deal. A course of treatments every few weeks is recommended, but you can have the odd treatment as needed.

Costs

£80–150 per treatment.

NIP TIP
Avoid having any resurfacing treatments (peels, microdermabrasion, light, lasers) if you have open sores, infections, a recent tan, or have taken Roaccutane® (a potent drug for cystic acne) for the past six months, without your doctor's permission.

LASERS AND LIGHT DEVICES

With laser treatments, it can be a bit hit and miss as to who gets a great result and who doesn't because of variables such as the condition of your skin, the type of laser used, the skill level of the physician and the number of treatments received. Most lasers and light devices target red or brown or both red and brown bits. Add to that their novel ability to tighten collagen and you have a wide spectrum of systems that can make dramatic improvements in your skin. Lasers are also not for faces only: they can treat what are known as 'off face' areas too – arms, legs, hands, chest and any other body part on your hit list.

Until recently, there were only two basic categories of laser treatment: ablative resurfacing and non-ablative laser or light-based therapy. Fractional lasers turned up and then there were three. Each has its own advantages and disadvantages.

Ablative lasers can regenerate ageing and sun-damaged skin, but have significant side effects and risks, cause prolonged redness and need prolonged recovery time. The gold standard of ablative or deep lasers is the carbon dioxide (CO_2). Lighter, non-ablative techniques such as IPLs generally carry fewer risks but require a course of treatments over several months and sometimes offer less dramatic results. Fractional lasers offer a slightly different twist – falling somewhere in between.

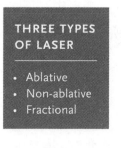

THREE TYPES OF LASER

- Ablative
- Non-ablative
- Fractional

Non-ablative lasers pass through the skin without vaporising it, so they don't burn the skin. They work beneath the surface skin layer to stimulate collagen growth and improve skin texture and tone. These devices heat tissue to different degrees of depth. They can deal with blood vessels or brown spots, and some of them can do a little collagen tightening. Lasers and laser-like devices have come down in power so that they cause less trauma and time out of commission; however, they require more than one go. Your choice is to do one big treatment or have a series of smaller treatments that may add up to the same result.

Most devices on offer today are not actually lasers. They have variations of energy that are delivered into the skin in different ways. Lasers that target the top layer of skin have been the primary treatment to reduce wrinkles and acne scarring. But they caused redness and messy oozing and needed long recuperation time. New techniques such as portrait plasma and fractional resurfacing are changing the way doctors approach skin resurfacing by regenerating the skin below the surface to increase results while decreasing downtime.

Getting started early can delay the signs of ageing and sun damage. Early intervention using laser, light, radio frequency and other non-invasive therapies can definitely help maintain a youthful, smooth-skinned appearance. If you have signs of ageing, can't take time out and don't need or want a facelift, but would like something to refresh and refine your skin, the newest crop of skin tightening and resurfacing systems could be just the ticket for you.

Intense Pulsed Light therapy (IPL)

IPL is the gold standard in photorejuvenation. The versatility of these devices has made them the workhorse in every cosmetic clinic; they treat many skin concerns at once such as brown spots, red veins, texture, tone, acne and unwanted hair. IPL uses broad-spectrum light to reverse the effects of ageing and sun damage on the face, neck, chest and even hands. IPL is exactly what it sounds like: intense light. It differs from a laser – which utilises coherent light of a single colour or wavelength – by using light that is neither coherent nor of a single wavelength. Different wavelengths of light interact with the skin in different ways. To treat red discolourations (such as thread veins or rosacea), light or laser absorbed by the red found within the blood vessels works best. Freckles, brown spots and unwanted hair may all be treated with light of a particular colour. Skin tightening happens with lights that tighten the collagen and elastin fibres by gently heating them. The levels of energy can be tailored to your specific needs. Results are modest, and you can expect to do these treatments fairly often to keep them up.

The procedure

A cold gel is usually applied to the areas to be treated and protective eyewear is worn. The surface of the handpiece is applied to your skin and light is delivered in precise pulses. You may feel a little sting like a rubber band being snapped against your skin.

Recovery time

Virtually no downtime; brief slight redness.

Risks

Darker skin types are more at risk of dark or light patches, scars and blotches; IPL treatments are safe if the technician is properly trained.

How long it lasts

Usually needs to be done in a series of three or more treatments to see visible improvements. Deeper lasers may zap a brown spot in just one go.

Costs

Fees vary by device and range from £200 to £500 per area per treatment.

Manufacturer

These are some companies that are well respected: www.lumenis.com, www.palomarmedical.com, www.cutera.com, www.syneron.com. There are many others.

> ### Angelika battles her brown spots
> **Sick of covering up a brown patch the size of a pea below her left eye, Angelika decided to do something about it. The beauty therapist who did her facials offered to use a light to take it away and**

> Angelika agreed. Straight away, she knew that something had gone horribly wrong. She felt an intense burn and got a blister. She swore she could see sparks fly! The therapist was bewildered. Weeks later, the brown spot was still there, and where the blister had burst she had a new red mark on top of it. Angelika was not pleased, and ended up spending another £500 to get it sorted by a proper laser clinic. The moral of this story is that any device that applies heat to the skin can cause a burn, and if you don't go to someone who is trained, there are always risks.

LED photorejuvenation

LED devices are becoming more compact and portable. The next generation will be suitable to use at home, enabling people to bypass the frequent visits to the clinic or salon needed to complete a course of treatments.

The procedure

Light emitting diode (LED) light sources are light therapy systems that deliver a low dosage of light (only 25 watts). The treatment consists of twice-a-week sessions lasting less than one minute for four weeks, followed by a booster session every month. Skin exfoliation with a peel or microdermabrasion is recommended before treatment. LEDs are also used with IPL treatments and toxin and filler injections to calm redness and swelling. The treatment helps sun damage and acne, but don't expect to be amazed; not everyone gets a dramatic improvement.

Recovery time

No discomfort and no downtime.

Risks

Virtually none.

How long it lasts

Multiple treatments are needed on an ongoing basis; this is not for someone who has limited free time.

Costs

Less than £80 per treatment.

Manufacturer

(GentleWaves®) Light Bioscience, US, www.lightbioscience.com; (Omnilux®, Lumiere Light Therapie) PhotoTherapeutics Ltd, UK, www.phototherapeutics.com.

Photo Pneumatic therapy

The procedure

Photo Pneumatic (PPx) therapy uses a combination of pressure and broadband light to treat the skin. The device draws the skin to be treated into the handpiece, and light energy converts to heat energy. This works for acne, sun damage and redness.

Recovery time

No discomfort and no downtime.

Risks

Virtually none: this is a very gentle treatment.

How long it lasts

Multiple sessions are needed, as with all light devices.

Costs

£200 per treatment.

Manufacturer

Aesthera, US, www.aesthera.com.

Photodynamic therapy (PDT)

The procedure

This is a two-stage treatment – first a solution is applied to the skin, and then a light activates it. Photodynamic therapy (PDT) marries the uses of a strong light or laser with a chemical that absorbs this energy when applied to the skin. It is used for acne, sun damage, enlarged pores, age spots and pre-cancerous lesions. PDT works when the light interacts with the dye that has been applied to the skin. The skin is cleansed with alcohol to allow the photosensitising agent to penetrate. The dye is allowed to penetrate the skin, and the skin is then treated with a BluLight, IPL or Pulsed Dye laser.

Recovery time

Some itching, burning or peeling, and redness comparable to sunburn.

Risks

Avoid the sun after the dye has been applied to your skin because it reacts with any light.

How long it lasts

Long-lasting results; may be repeated as needed.

Costs

Comparable to other non-ablative laser and light treatments.

Manufacturer

DUSA Pharmaceuticals Inc., US, www.levulan.com.

Fractional lasers

The hottest resurfacing devices fall within this fairly new category. There are many systems now that can produce fractionated results. Fraxel® was the first of these to be introduced.

The procedure

Fraxel® laser treatment requires some topical anaesthestic or numbing cream, as it is very uncomfortable (similar to Thermage®). The cooling device helps a lot by frosting the skin with arctic air. The results are good for pigment, melasma, skin tone and texture, and mild acne scars; but the treatment is not intended for deep wrinkles. One advantage of this technology is that it can be used to treat the neck, chest, arms, hands and legs.

Recovery time

Expect a mild sunburn effect for about an hour afterwards. Swelling and redness generally settle down in three days. The skin may remain pink for about a week, and feels tight and dry.

Risks

Some of the risks of other lasers, including skin lightening, darkening and scarring, but these are quite rare.

How long it lasts

Three to four treatments are needed, and results are considered long lasting, but maintenance is needed. It takes several months to see the full effect.

Costs

About £1,000 per area per treatment.

Manufacturer

Reliant Technologies, US, www.fraxel.com.

Plasma skin regeneration

Portrait® plasma skin regeneration is another newcomer. The Portrait® PSR3 System deposits nitrogen plasma energy into the skin without damaging the surface. It preserves the skin's outer layers, which act as a protective dressing until new skin generates. The goal is to get better results than those from non-ablative treatments, while producing a tightening effect equivalent to a single pass by full-on lasers such as carbon dioxide. It is used to reduce wrinkles, improve skin tone, texture and elasticity, reduce brown spots and pore size, and tighten skin.

The procedure

The energy is applied directly to the skin's surface. Ionised plasma delivers energy to where the plasma gives up energy upon tissue contact. The device is versatile; you can have multiple very low-energy treatments, called Portrait Express®, or a single high-energy treatment. Higher energies will give better results, with a longer recovery. The system is considered to offer a full spectrum of treatments from the equivalent of a chemical peel to a single-pass deep-laser resurfacing technique. A full-face high-energy treatment takes about ten minutes; a full-face very low-energy treatment takes 10 minutes.

Recovery time

A topical numbing cream is sufficient for the low-energy treatments; for high-energy treatments you may need pain pills or a local anaesthetic. Your skin remains intact for the first few days until it begins to peel when the new epidermis has formed. There will be some redness and swelling for a week after a high-energy treatment.

Risks

Redness and flaking should be expected; the treatment is safer for lighter skin types, and currently not recommended for dark brown or black skin types.

How long it lasts

One or more treatments are generally done; results are long-lasting, and continue to improve for several months.

Costs

£1,000–2,000 per treatment.

Manufacturer

Rhytec, UK, www.rhytec.com.

SURFING THE WAVES

Compared with fillers, there are even more laser and light systems on the market. I have highlighted only some of the most popular devices from the major manufacturers. There are many other devices that can create the same or similar effect. Unless you are a physicist, you can't be expected to know which is the best technology for you – that is the job of the doctor you go to. Choose a doctor who uses several different systems and has experience with skin lasers. If a doctor uses only one

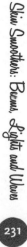

device, he is likely to try it on you, even though it may not be ideal for what you want.

DEVICE	skin rejuvenation	wrinkles	acne	red veins	brown spots	hair removal
ED	✓		✓			
Erbium:YAG	✓	✓				
Nd:YAG	✓	✓		✓	✓	✓
Pulsed light	✓			✓	✓	
Pulsed dye	✓			✓		
Q-Switched Ruby	✓			✓	✓	
Diode	✓			✓		
Alexandrite	✓			✓	✓	

WHAT TO KNOW BEFORE YOU GET LASERED

- What is the name of the technology?
- Is this the best technology to accomplish my goals?
- How long has it been on the market?
- How long has the doctor been using it?
- What is the name of the manufacturer and where are they located?
- What kinds of clinical studies have been done?
- What are the possible side-effects?
- What does a reaction look like and how long does it last?
- What can be done if I have a reaction?
- How many treatments will I need and how often?
- How much will each treatment cost?
- If it doesn't look right, what can be done?
- Can I still have other lasers and treatments later on?
- Does it have a CE mark?
- Is it FDA approved?
- Is the manufacturer planning to apply for FDA approval in the near future?

Après lasers

New skin needs special care. After any type of laser or light therapy, your skin will be very sensitive to UV light, and may react to anything.

Don't

- Apply any acids to your skin: alpha hydroxy, beta hydroxy, lactic, Retin-A®, etc.
- Get direct sun exposure for three to six weeks.
- Use abrasive scrubs, exfoliants or gommages; these should be avoided until you are no longer red.

Do

Post-lasered skin needs TLC. Petrolatum products (such as that used for nappy rash) can double up to promote healing and prevent crusting. Ask your pharmacist or try the following.

- **Catrix® 10 Ointment** Intensive petrolatum-based healing agent. See www.catrix.com.
- **Skinceuticals Phyto Corrective Gel** Soothing anti-inflammatory botanical gel with a fresh herbal scent. See www.skinceuticals.co.uk.
- **Skin Medica® TNS Recovery Complex** Cult favourite in America for post-laser peelings. See www.skinbrands.co.uk.

SKIN TIGHTENING SANS SCALPEL

The trendy names for the latest wave of facial rejuvenation treatments make them sound very posh, and procedures promoted as lift alternatives strike a special chord among women who can't or won't have real surgery. It all adds up to a growing number of women who are eager to bypass traditional facelifts in favour of a slew of state-of-the-art advances in non-invasive techniques.

These high-tech skin-tightening devices use a handheld instrument to transmit energy through the skin to heat the collagen fibres in the dermis, causing them to contract and tighten. Although nothing like a facelift, these procedures can subtly improve early skin slackening on the jowls and neck.

Thermage®, the first of these, uses radio-frequency technology, something that has been used in medicine for years. A handheld device directs radio waves deep within the skin, where they cause tissue to heat as well as some structural alterations (the skin's surface is cooled by a spray to prevent burning and to make the procedure more comfortable). The skin tightens as the collagen contracts and it can continue to do so for up to six months. Since the skin surface is not treated, you can look presentable within a few hours. Not everyone gets the same effect and it doesn't always work. If you don't see enough of a result after one session, you can have another go.

At best, the lifting effect is pretty modest compared to a surgical lift; for example, your brows may be lifted by about two or three millimetres. This translates into a fresher, brighter look rather than a dramatically younger appearance. Skin-tightening technologies all do something to generally shrink skin in a slightly different way. Extra treatments produce better results. As with so many other cosmetic procedures, not every technician gets the same results. Because of the subtlety factor, it works best if you are in your late thirties or forties and are only beginning to show signs of facial sag, although older women have also benefited. You can still get improvement in your fifties and sixties, but collagen building takes longer.

Discomfort is a definite consideration. Most people consider skin tightening worse than laser hair removal and not as bad as a bunionectomy. The continuous spray of cooling is mandatory to keep you comfortable. The amount of pain also has a lot to do with who is doing the treatment. If the practitioner goes slowly and takes breaks between zaps, it takes longer but hurts less.

There are many technologies on the market and, as you would guess, new ones popping up every day. Each new device promises to be faster, better and lower on the pain scale. Radio-frequency devices come in unipolar (Thermage®) or bipolar (Aluma™) as a means of delivering the energy. Unipolar means that there is one source; bipolar means there are two. The Titan® system uses infrared energy, not radio waves, to renew elasticity. Generally, the more tightening you need or want, the more sessions will be necessary.

Skin-tightening treatments are quickly gaining popularity for any part of the body with wrinkly skin where a few millimetres of shrinkage would be a welcome benefit. In rank order of request, the most favoured body areas to have treated are the tummy, thighs and upper arms. For bigger areas, several treatments are usually necessary and each session may take hours to have done. For example, to Titan® a tummy may take two or more hours, the face and neck about an hour. Post-pregnancy, it can be great for smoothing crinkly bits of skin around your tummy button. The good news is that main body parts sting less than delicate eyelids, cheeks and chins.

Once significant droop has set in, the only reliable way to reverse it is a proper lift of some sort. These treatments are not always a home run. You have to be realistic – they are capable of only subtle alterations – but the skin takes on a smoothness, radiance and bounciness. If you go into it expecting a steak dinner, you will be disappointed – you're probably only going to get hors d'oeuvres.

Thermage®

The procedure

Thermage® uses a computer to create a layer of radio-frequency energy with a consistent shape that is delivered to a particular location on the skin. Multiple passes are made over each area to be treated in order to super-heat the dermal layer, causing it to contract and tighten. First used for the face and neck, Thermage® is now used for crêpey thighs, loose tummies, sagging arms and ageing hands. It can also help with décolleté lines and creases. Most people describe it as moderately painful.

Recovery time

There is no downtime.

Risks

Considered a safe technique; however, if it is not done properly the underlying fat can be altered, which can result in irregularities and scarring.

How long it lasts

The tightening effects are immediate and improve over time for about 12 months.

Costs

About £3,000 for a full-face and neck treatment.

Manufacturer

Thermage, US, www.thermage.com.

Titan®

The procedure

Titan® utilises infrared light to heat deep tissues beneath the skin's surface to produce younger, springier skin. It smoothes out crêpey, textured skin on the face and the body. The Titan® XL spot size is twice as large as the original Titan®, so it takes less time and covers more ground, so to speak. It can achieve some lifting effect and reduction in wrinkles and acne, and tightening in areas of the body such as loose tummies, saggy breasts, and droopy upper arms and inner thighs.

Recovery time

With each pulse, you feel a brief heating sensation, followed by the frost of the skin-cooling system which reduces stinging. Tightening effects are instant in most cases, and there is no down time. The effect of new collagen development appears gradually over a few months.

Risks

The biggest risk is that you don't get enough of a result.

How long it lasts

The skin-tightening results are said to last one to two years.

Costs

Fees range from £1,000 to £2,000 per treatment. Usually two to three treatments are needed per area.

Manufacturer

Cutera, US, www.cutera.com.

ReFirme™

The procedure

The ReFirme™ ST Applicator is designed for skin tightening and rejuvenation, but works slightly differently from its predecessors. The system combines pulses of infrared light simultaneously with bipolar radio frequency.

Recovery time

Virtually no downtime; slight redness may occur.

Risks

Results are variable, as with all skin-tightening devices.

How long it lasts

Maintenance treatments are needed after about 12–18 months.

Costs

Fees range, from £250 per area per treatment.

Manufacturer

Syneron, Israel, www.syneron.com.

Aluma™

The procedure

This radio-frequency technology is delivered by using a handpiece that serves as a vacuum to tighten the skin and deliver heat directly to the deeper layers. It regenerates collagen, which is necessary to maintain skin firmness and reduce wrinkles.

Recovery time

The procedure takes about 15 minutes, after which you may resume normal activities.

Risks

Low risk and virtually pain-free.

How long it lasts

Multiple treatments are needed; ongoing maintenance is suggested.

Costs

From £200 per area per treatment.

Manufacturer

Lumenis, Israel, www.aesthetic.lumenis.com.

CELLULITE SOLUTIONS

Nothing says 'adorable' like a cute pair of dimples in your cheeks. But when dimples turn up on your thighs and buttocks, there is nothing cute about them. The problem is cellulite, annoying dents and divets that can appear on even the skinniest body.

Cellulite is not a fat problem: it's a skin problem. It doesn't correlate to how much you weigh. The fat that causes cellulite is not the same as the fat that takes you from a size 8 to a 12. Cellulite is made up of fat cells that live deep within the skin and are not burned as fuel. Nothing really targets cellulite – not starvation diets, rigorous exercise or even liposuction. Cellulite is a decidedly female problem, which indicates that hormones are involved somewhere along the line. It's genetic, too, passed down like a family heirloom of the kind that gets tucked away in a safety deposit box in a bank in the Midlands somewhere.

For generations, doctors claimed that cellulite was a figment of our imagination. Most women at one time or another have raised their hands in frustration, and accepted it as our lumpy, bumpy plight. But in the last few years several promising treatment options have emerged. Some women see a difference, or maybe they just want desperately to believe that their thighs are smoother than they were before they spent a small fortune. The science is still a bit shaky, but these treatments are worth a closer look.

One development is the use of light energy to melt cellulite while mechanically massaging the skin to increase circulation and encourage drainage of lymph vessels. TriActive® Laser Dermology relies on laser light. It works by first cooling the skin so that the laser can penetrate

Skin Smoothers: Beams, Lights and Waves

deep without harming the top layer and then using a combination of suction and energy to treat the cellulite. The device increases circulation on a cellular level, removing fluids and putting pressure on fat cells, while the suction supposedly loosens the septa bands to diminish the dimpling effect. See www.cynosure.com.

Another of these light devices, VelaSmooth®, uses a combination of radio-frequency energy and infrared light to heat up and then release cellulite from cells. At the same time, it rolls over skin in a massaging motion, using suction to soften and release septa bands. See www.syneron.com.

Endermologie®, a hi-tech massage from France (where else?), has been around for decades. It is basically deep mechanically assisted lymphatic drainage that combines rollers and suction to attack connective tissue, stimulate blood flow and drain fluids. Although it feels very invigorating, results are pretty temporary and compliance is a problem. Who really has the time to trek all over town to have a 45-minute session twice a week? See www.lpgone.com.

Thinner thighs don't come cheap or fast. These systems require multiple sessions spread out over time, and the cost will run well into the thousands. And if you do get any results, they may last six months or longer, but maintenance treatments will be needed to keep dimples at bay.

Cellulite is primarily a young woman's nemesis. When the rest of your body is tight and firm, and looks good naked, rippled patches spoil an otherwise perfect and smooth plane. However, add a decade or two and a couple of kids, and your perspective changes. How do you decide which bothers you most? Is it your lines and wrinkles, a saggy bottom or the waddle under your chin that makes you mad? In comparison, the odd dimple might not be all that important, especially if you cover it up anyway.

GUNS AND NEEDLES

Among the most controversial non-surgical treatments is the category called mesotherapy. Developed in France in the 1950s, this involves injections of a mixture of medicines combined with vitamins, herbs and anaesthetics reminiscent of the bubbly broth mixed by the three witches in *Macbeth*. The cocktail (which can vary widely among practitioners) is administered in a series of rapid injections into the mesoderm, or middle layer of skin. It is a mainstay along the Mediterranean in France, Spain, Italy and Greece. The needles are teeny, like a cross between those used for acupuncture and Botox®, and you need a lot of them to do the job.

The process begins by applying a numbing cream to the skin. While it takes effect, syringes containing a nutrient supplement called phosphatidylcholine, which comes from soybeans, is mixed with a bio-salt solution, which is known to dissolve and digest fat.

To get a uniform result, a washable ink grid pattern is applied to your skin. Dozens of small injections of the solution are made along the grid's precise pattern. Next you are subjected to a few minutes with an ultrasound wand that helps to distribute the solution evenly within the fat cells. Only small areas can be treated, so this is not a weight-loss tool. Once the fat cells are gone, they will never come back – which is similar to the way liposuction works.

This method can be used for fatty tumours, pot bellies, saddlebags, eyebags and jowly blobs. Treatment involves a series of multiple injections, from five for the neck to 25 or more for a larger body area, spaced four to six weeks apart, during which time fat continues to dissolve. To keep the dissolving action of the solution within the layer of fat cells, the needles used are adjusted to very specific lengths. The injections are not fun and may leave temporary needle marks. Some swelling is to be expected, especially for the face and tummy, so there is a healing process even if it doesn't last too long. A session will cost around £350–500 and multiple treatments per area are required.

Injectable fat-dissolving cocktails go by the names Lipodissolve®, Lipomelt®, FlabJab® and numerous other quirky-sounding names. The problem is that they are not licensed in most countries, including the UK and the US, so clinics do these treatments under the radar of the local health authorities.

Although it sounds like junk science because it seems too good to be true, many women and their doctors swear by this treatment. There is clinical evidence that phosphatidylcholine does something to fat and cellulite, and perhaps in the very near future we can expect to witness a turning point. There are many studies under way in various parts of the world, being conducted both by long-time mesotherapists eager to prove the validity of their methods, and sceptics curious about the mechanism of the action. This technique works and it is likely to be legitimised very soon.

BIO-REVITALISATION

In France, this technique – often referred to as mesolifting – uses hyaluronic acid and vitamins to rejuvenate the face. Hyaluronic acid is used in a different manner from fillers by hydrating, restructuring and rejuvenating tired, ageing, damaged-looking skin, improving its elasticity and tone. Some of these injectable mixtures also claim to increase the production of fibroblasts, the forerunners to collagen and elastin. A session every fortnight for at least two months is recommended, then maintenance treatments every two to four months.

There are many brands of hyaluronic acid on the market including Elastence®, Restylane® Vital, Teosyal® Kiss, Hyal-System® and about a gazillion others. Doctors touting this method also tend to mix their own concoctions, which vary tremendously. You have to be Sherlock Holmes's much younger sister to decipher what is in these mixtures, and results are inconsistent from clinic to clinic.

Ask The Beauty Junkie®

How can you tell if a laser is safe?

New devices pop up on the market about every two years with all sorts of enticing claims that compare them to facelifts and tummy tucks. Technology is being launched at lightning speed, and there is a lot of pressure to get to market quickly. Devices often get introduced to the consumer before the doctors have had a chance to evaluate properly their safety and effectiveness. The FDA approves devices as 'safe and effective', but that is no guarantee that any system really works better than something else that is already available. A CE mark is required for a medical device to be marketed in Europe; however, this is the same mark that is given to common kitchen appliances, such as the toaster you use to make your breakfast.

What is the difference between a peel and microdermabrasion?

Chemical peels can achieve an even shedding of damaged skin cells. A solution is applied to the skin to remove dead skin cells and stimulate the production of new cells. There are many solutions used in varying concentrations from superficial to much deeper peeling.

Microdermabrasion has a similar effect on the skin; however, it uses tiny particles to slough the outermost layer of the skin. The treatment may be altered by adjusting the depth of the sanding.

What is the difference between microdermabrasion and dermabrasion?

Microdermabrasion blasts the skin with sterile microparticles to abrade or rub off the top layer, and then vacuums out the particles and the dead skin. Microdermabrasion alone is not ideal for treating wrinkles and brown spots; it enhances the penetration of topical medicines to treat ageing or acne. It can be used to refine texture and tone and to smooth superficial lines. Dermabrasion is a mechanical sanding of the skin using a handheld rotary instrument with a fine wheel (called a fraise). It is more aggressive than micro-dermabrasion, and rarely used any more since the advent of lasers.

Are the sutures used for threadlifts permanent?

Some threads are designed to remain permanently; however, other resorbable models are currently undergoing clinical investigation and are expected to be launched very soon. These sutures will dissolve within 6 to 12 months, and hopefully will retain most of their holding strength.

Will lasers leave you permanently red?

Fortunately, most of the devices used today are not technically lasers, but variations of light and heat energy that work in different ways. It's no longer a fire zone, but many systems will cause a temporary pink or reddish colouring on your skin. In some cases you can see a line of demarcation where the treatment ended, which blends over time.

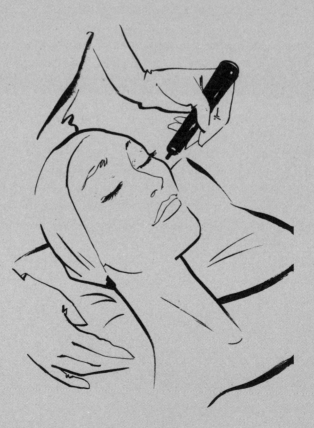

11

Bits and Pieces

You know those little niggling bits and flaws that show up out of nowhere on your skin? You don't have to live with them if you don't want to. In New York and LA, it is de rigueur to pop into your dermatologist once or twice a year for a simple clinical clean-up of moles, skin tags, veiny things and the occasional freckle.

COMMON BEAUTY AFFLICTIONS

Open pores

Pores expand because they become clogged with dead cells and oil, which make them look larger. Sun damage, lack of exfoliation and clogging blackheads are common culprits.

What is the remedy?

To get pores back to their normal size, you need to get rid of the blockage that caused them to expand. The key elements are unplugging the pores and cleaning away dirt, bacteria and oil; limiting sun exposure; exfoliating; and using the right ingredients such vitamin A, azelaic acid, and alpha and beta hydroxy acids.

Moles

As moles age, the pigment gets deeper, so they lose their colour and stick out more, which makes them more visible.

What is the remedy?

A simple shave biopsy can bring the mole down to the level of the surrounding skin. If this is done right, it doesn't even leave a scar. Moles can also be excised, but then a scar is a given.

Skin tags

A skin tag is a bit of skin that sticks out and may appear attached to the skin. It may be smooth or irregular, flesh coloured or pigmented, raised or dangling. Skin tags can show up almost anywhere, but most commonly appear on the eyelids, neck, armpits and chest, and especially in women.

What is the remedy?

They can be instantly snipped away almost painlessly with surgical scissors.

Seborrheic keratoses

Called 'barnacles of old age', these benign lesions are caused by excessive growth of the top layer of skin cells. They show up on the body, under the breasts, on shoulders and in places where they get rubbed by clothing. They can range from light tan to black in colour, and look as if they have been pasted on your skin.

What is the remedy?

Electrocautery or hot iron tip can be used to melt these right off. Carbon dioxide laser is also useful.

Dermatoses papulosa nigra

These are little black or dark brown bumps that usually appear on dark skin, and start out as little freckles under the eyes and on the top of the cheekbones. They can grow in clusters, and tend to run in families.

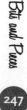

What is the remedy?

Electrocautery or hot iron tip can be used to melt these right off.

Xantholasma

These yellowish fatty or cholesterol deposits tend to show up around the eyelids.

What is the remedy?

Carbon dioxide lasers can melt them away. They can also be excised if they are really deep, but this can leave a small scar.

Eccrine spiradenoma

These are little flesh-toned bumps that appear under the eyelids.

What is the remedy?

Electrocautery or hot iron tip can be used to melt these right off. Lasers also work.

Sebaceous hyperplasia

These are enlarged sebaceous glands with a pore that looks like a pit in the middle. They are often yellowish, soft and rounded. They usually show up on the forehead, cheeks and nose, or areas of the face that have a large concentration of oil glands.

What is the remedy?

Electrocautery or hot iron tip can be used to melt these right off. Lasers can also be used to get rid of them.

Thread veins

Spider veins or telangiectasias are commonly found around the nose and on cheeks, legs and the chest, though they can appear almost anywhere. They are small, super-fine capillaries that lie close to the skin's surface. They can show up as a true spider shape with a squiggly mass of capillaries radiating out from a dark centre, resemble tiny branches or appear as thin separate lines. They are more common in women, especially when oestrogen levels rise.

What is the remedy?

Vascular lasers and light sources cause tiny veins to collapse; electrocautery is sometimes used. For leg veins, sclerotherapy injections are also used, in which a solution is injected into the veins, causing them to collapse.

Milia

These are clogged ducts or teeny sebaceous cysts on the face. Milia can show up around the eyes, on cheekbones and on the forehead. Over-moisturising or using too creamy products can be the culprit. Sun damage and laser treatments are also possible causes.

What is the remedy?

Your doctor may use a small needle or blade to pluck out the glob of thickened oil. Milia can be treated by extraction, and microdermabrasion and peels can also help.

Shaving bumps

Called pseudo-folliculitis barbae, shaving bumps are a widespread problem, especially among women with curly hair and in the bikini

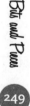

area and underarms. As the hair follicle grows out of the skin, it immediately curls and re-enters the skin. The skin becomes inflamed and irritated, creating bumps.

What is the remedy?

Wash the area twice daily with an exfoliant to raise the hairs from under the skin and prevent them from growing back into the skin. Bumps can also be relieved by using glycolic acid lotions, antibiotic gels and Retin-A®. Other options include laser treatments to remove the hair follicles.

Keratosis pilaris

A genetic condition of the follicles that sometimes resembles acne, but appears as rough bumps on the upper arms, backs of the thighs and buttocks. It is also common in teens.

What is the remedy?

Common remedies include exfoliating, moisturising and using Retin-A® or an alpha hydroxy acid. Avoid scratching the bumps, as this may lead to scarring or spreading.

Poikiloderma

Excessively pigmented areas (brownish, reddish), particularly on the chest and neck, caused by long-term sun exposure.

What is the remedy?

Lasers can target the blood vessels and clear up the spotty appearance of skin.

Redness and rosacea

Redness, or rosacea, is actually a sign of ageing and skin thinning. Tiny red veins peek through the skin and create blushing. The hallmark of rosacea, also called the curse of the Celts, is facial flushing in response to sun exposure, red wine, spices, smoking and steam heat. The origin is often related to the blood vessels; most people have some broken capillaries and redness around the nose, cheeks and chin. Hormones play a role in rosacea, and flare-ups are more likely during your monthly period or with menopause.

What is the remedy?

The most common treatments for rosacea include topical antibiotics and oral medications. Pulsed dye laser and intense pulsed light are the gold standard for zapping the redness of rosacea. The pulsed dye laser is good for thicker blood vessels, while intense pulsed light treatments work nicely for fine vessels. No topical vitamin K cream can visibly shrink a capillary, but it may reduce redness. See also Flushing and Blushing section.

Age spots

They may be called freckles when you are young, and some people think they are cute, but in your forties they appear as dark brown patches. They are caused by sun exposure.

What is the remedy?

Age spots on the face or hands can be treated with bleaching agents, peels and lasers. Hydroquinone is a doctor's staple for lightening excessively pigmented skin, but it is not on the market in the UK. Koijic acid is an alternative skin lightener derived from a Japanese mushroom that is usually used in combination with other ingredients. Microdermabrasion and chemical peels uncover a fresh layer of skin; glycolic and salicylic acids exfoliate, which helps lightening agents penetrate better.

Stretch marks

After skin has been stretched by rapid growth due to pregnancy, weight gain or loss, stretch marks, or striae, can show up, often starting as reddish or purplish in colour, then taking on a shiny appearance, streaked in silver or white. Stretch marks occur in the dermis, the elastic middle layer of skin that allows it to retain its shape, which stretches like a rubber band. Women can get stretch marks on the tummy area, thighs, hips, breasts, upper arms or lower back.

What is the remedy?

Stretch marks are basically just another form of scars. They appear show up in at least half of all pregnant women, usually in the later half of pregnancy, on the lower abdomen, thighs, hips, buttocks, breasts and arms. Topical Retin-A or vitamin A derivatives are your first port of call. Next steps up would include collagen tightening lasers and light devices. Vitamin E oil, emu oil, cocoa butter and other emollients are frequently recommended for use during pregnancy to prevent stretch marks from forming. Lasers work by destroying the top layers of scarred skin and can lighten dark stretch mark or reduce redness. Silvery or whitened stretch marks are the most difficult to improve. Prevention methods, including exercising during pregnancy, keeping your weight stable throughout your life, and keeping skin well hydrated, can help stretch marks from showing up as pronounced.

Scars – shallow

Shallow scars resulting from acne and chicken pox give skin a wavy appearance.

What is the remedy?

Fillers for deeper scars. Resurfacing lasers and light devices are well suited to shallow scars. Combination therapy is often the most effective.

Scars – raised

Two major types of scars, hypertrophic (raised, red) and keloid (thickened, overgrown), appear most frequently in young people and darker skin types. While hypertrophic scars remain one size, keloids can continue to grow into benign tumours if left untreated. Scars last for ever, but they will fade on their own over time, and can definitely be improved.

What is the remedy?

Thanks to the refinement of several techniques, scars can be treated with a variety of procedures to minimise their appearance.

Excision and punch replacement graft A depressed scar is surgically removed and a patch of skin is grafted from elsewhere on the body.

Fillers Hyaluronic acid fillers, polymer implants or your own fat (taken from another part of the body) are injected in small quantities below the surface of the skin to elevate depressed scars.

Laser therapy By delivering short pulses, this can smooth out, sculpt and refine raised scars, and normalise pigment (red, pink, and brown).

Peeling By applying a solution, mild scarring and certain types of acne scars may be improved over time.

Microdermabrasion Microdermabrasion crystals remove the dead layer of cells. By adding more pressure and more suction, and increasing the flow of crystals, exfoliation can go deeper to help stimulate and restore collagen and the elastic fibres in the skin's deeper layer.

Dermabrasion The area is injected with local anaesthetic and the skin is removed with a rotary instrument. It undergoes a remodelling process as it heals, resulting in a smoother appearance.

Steroids Steroids are commonly injected to flatten raised scars. This should be done with care because too much may cause a depressed area.

BAD HAIR DAYS

If you find stray hairs on your pillow, in your brush or lining your bathroom sink, you are not alone. Any woman over 40 knows that she doesn't have as many hairs on her head as she did at the age of 20. Women tend to have an overall thinning, rather than a distinct pattern of hair loss, but that can happen too. Thinning at the temples and hairline is not uncommon, and after face- and browlift surgery, your hairline may be moved back (which can be a telltale sign of

NEW HOPE FOR HAIR LOSS

HairMax™ Laser Comb – this hand-held home device was FDA-cleared to promote hair growth in men. It uses low-level laser therapy to regrow hair. See www.lasercomb.net.

Plastic Makes Perfect

cosmetic surgery). Don't despair – transplants actually work well in women and can be used to fill in thinning spots.

The procedure

It works basically like planting a garden: hair is removed from one area and transferred to thinning areas. After initially falling out within two to three weeks, the transplanted hair regrows, approximately two to three months later, and will continue to grow in the new area for as long as it would have grown where it was before. It also has the same colour and texture as the hair in the donor area. Follicular units are obtained by sectioning a fine strip of skin, usually from the back of the scalp. In a single session, several areas can be filled in to look very natural. Small incisions are made in the same direction that the hair grows in, and the grafts are carefully transferred into those sites. A fine scar remains at the donor site, and the same scar can be used for subsequent transplants. A new technique called Follicular Unit Extraction (FUE) bypasses the need for the removal of a strip from the donor area. A tiny round punch is used to excise each individual follicular unit, so it has the advantage of avoiding a scar, which makes it possible to harvest hair from other places.

NIP TIP
Losing your lashes? Follicular Unit Extraction may be used for individual transplants on lashes and brows too. Jan Marini Age Intervention® Eyelash is a brush-on formula for fluffing up lashes – see www.janmarini.com. Or try Osmotics FNS Nutrilash Lash and Brow Enhancer – see www.osmotics.com.

Post-op effects and recovery time

Initially, there are small crusts on the recipient sites. These fall off within three to ten days. Post-op pain is controllable with medication for the first one or two nights. Temporary swelling of the forehead usually lasts for about one week.

Risks

Bleeding or infection are always possible. If the grafts are not handled

Bits and Pieces

properly, if too many are transferred during a single session or if the grafts are planted too densely, some of the transplanted hairs may not grow.

Time in operating theatre

Three to six hours.

Minimum spend

£3,000–6,000. To find a qualified hair restoration surgeon, visit www.ishrs.org.

GRIN AND BARE IT

Laser hair removal is to shaving your legs what laser eye surgery is to wearing glasses – pure unadulterated freedom! Smooth skin can be yours with ease, especially with the new systems on offer. The laser beam or light pulse destroys the hair bulb itself. At least three sessions are needed to get long-term, and in some cases, permanent hair removal. Even after several treatments, you may have some stray hairs sneaking back, but they will be finer and usually lighter in colour.

Laser or light systems can be used anywhere hair may appear, even places you may never have thought of such as toes and nipples. Underarms, forearms, bikini area, and upper and lower legs are the standard. If you are tempted to sculpt or go bare down there, laser devices avoid the sting and irritating stubble between waxings. Laser hair removal may also be used by Polycystic Ovarian Syndrome (PCOS) sufferers, who may experience frustrating facial hair growth (and sadly often hair loss on their heads). The upper lip and chin growth and Elvis-like sideburns that can creep up on women can also be gone for good. Even a unibrow (think Frieda Kahlo) is fair game for lasers.

Risks include blistering, which may cause skin lightening or darkening, scarring and infections, which are rare. Thick, coarse or curly hair may require more treatments than soft, fine, lighter hair. As with any heat-activated treatment, darker skin is always at greater risk of discolouration. For dark brown and black skin, ask for a test on your forearm or inner thigh to make sure the system and setting are right for your skin. If you get little red bumps after hair removal (called folliculitis) ask your doctor for an antibiotic cream. Be careful about applying topical numbing cream or gel without medical supervision – very high levels of absorption can cause death.

NIP TIP
To slow facial hair regrowth in between treatments, Vaniqa® (Eflornithine Hydrochloride) cream is available on prescription. See www.vaniqa.com.

Technological advances have produced a more uniform application of light energy and more success in treating a wider range of skin and hair types.

Melanin-targeting lasers Ruby, alexandrite and flashlamp provide a wavelength of light that is absorbed by melanin. They are most effective on light skin with dark hair. With dark skin, normal skin pigment may be damaged.

Ruby lasers Designed to deliver maximum light energy to the follicle with minimum impact on the skin's surface. There are some risks of short-term loss of skin colour and blistering. This treatment works best on light skin and dark hair. If you have fair or light-coloured hair, it may not do the trick.

Alexandrite lasers In addition to melanin, these lasers allow absorption by haemoglobin (a red pigment in the red blood cells).

Flashlamp lasers This method applies a broad band of energy directly to the tissue, generated by a flashlamp rather than a single wavelength of a laser.

Nd:YAG Utilises a carbon-based cream to loosen hair from the follicle. It was the first type of laser to be FDA-approved for hair removal.

HAND REJUVENATION

Your face is tight as a drum, but what about those old-lady hands? Your hands take a lot of abuse. They are subjected to cumulative sun exposure and collagen breakdown, just as the face is. The skin on the hands also tends to be thin, and sun damage causes brown spots, slackening and wrinkling. Wear a hand cream with SPF 15 or higher daily.

Bits and Pieces

What is the remedy?

- chemical peels
- IPL treatments
- Thermage®
- Q-switched Nd: YAG
- Fraxel®
- Restylane® Vital
- fat injections

SMILE REDESIGN

Having a great smile sends a signal to the world that you are confident, attractive, desirable and even smart. Each of us has a natural smile style, based on the natural neuromuscular patterns we are born with. For example, some people show only their upper teeth when they smile, whereas others raise and lower their lips at the same time, revealing all their upper and lower teeth.

From an aesthetic perspective, a gorgeous smile has the power to disarm, charm and awe everyone with whom you come in contact, and it is often the first feature people notice when they meet you. Many of us hesitate to open wide and bear our pearly whites, simply because we feel the pearliness isn't quite up to par. Every effort made to avoid showing your smile – a cleverly placed hand or a tense smile beneath tightly pursed lips – makes this insecurity even more apparent.

Even a perfect smile deteriorates as we get older. Your teeth naturally wear down, gums recede and teeth become darker and more dis-coloured. As the face ages, lips lose muscle tone and begin to sag, revealing more of the lower teeth. Years of use (eating abrasive foods, brushing teeth, and natural wear and tear) erode the enamel of the teeth along the biting edges. The edges of the upper teeth wear down and teeth appear shorter from grinding. With age, the teeth may start to lean in because there is less to support the muscle structure.

While many people are dissatisfied with their smiles, only a small percentage of people actually realise how simple it is to change them.

Cosmetic dentists can give you the smile you used to have or the one you wish you were born with. The upper teeth can be lengthened with porcelain veneers, giving the lip better support and filling out lines and hollows around the mouth that have collapsed. The lower teeth can be contoured to make them appear shorter and more delicate.

The two basic options for rejuvenating your smile are whitening techniques, and customised porcelain veneers. A simple whitening procedure can take years off your face. Bleaching options are temporary, and may last one to two years. Porcelain veneers can transform your smile in just two visits and last one to two decades with good maintenance. Natural-looking veneers should have a radiant, translucent quality that complements your skin tone.

Lighten up

When it comes to teeth, no one ever thinks theirs are white enough. Some people naturally begin with teeth that have a yellowish hue, while others have noticed more recent discolouration from staining foods like coffee, red wine and colas. Bleaching agents work best on yellow or brown teeth and are not as effective on grey-colored stains caused by medications like antibiotics. If your teeth are extremely discoloured, veneers or bonding are the only way to go.

Most whitening toothpastes merely remove surface stains so they won't offer you a dramatic change. Results are superficial because the paste or gum only stays on teeth for a short time. As soon as you go back to your old habits of Starbuck's and cabernet, staining will return.

The results of in-office power bleaching offer a more long-lasting effect. A bleaching solution is applied directly to the tooth and is then exposed to a high intensity light, which accelerates the oxidation process. The oxygen travels into the inner layers of the teeth and dissolves the stained molecules, allowing more light to transmit through the teeth and make them look whiter. The alternative is a home bleaching kit that uses a customised mould filled with a carbamide peroxide gel, which fits over the teeth. The process usually takes several weeks of continuous use to work. Too much bleaching can make teeth more sensitive to hot and cold, but this is usually only temporary and reverses itself.

Tooth bonding

Bonding is the precursor to porcelain laminates or veneers. It may be useful for correcting broken or misshapen teeth, but is nowhere near as durable or as versatile as porcelain veneers. It is, however, considerably cheaper. Bonding is often used for chipped, stained or fractured teeth or to close the space between two teeth. The enamel layer of the tooth is etched with mildly acidic solution and a matching composite resin or plastic paste is moulded onto the teeth. The composite resin is hardened by a high-intensity light and then sculpted to reshape the teeth. The disadvantages of bonding are that it only lasts about three to six years, and it tends to discolour and chip.

Porcelain veneers

If your goal is a true smile redesign, the most effective long-term method is with expertly shaped porcelain veneers. This involves applying a thin veneer of preformed porcelain directly to tooth structure. At the first visit, the tooth structure is filed down to make room for the laminates. Thin layers of fine porcelain are then carefully fitted to improve the colour, shape, size and alignment of the teeth. Composite resin cement binds tooth surface to the porcelain securely. This procedure requires local anaesthestic and takes a few hours in the dentist's chair to complete.

The strength and beauty of porcelain and its translucent qualities provide a natural-looking appearance. Porcelain does not stain so your new smile will stay white for years to come. The end results are cosmetic restorations that are truly undetectable, yet incredibly mesmerising.

Straightening teeth

Braces used to be a rite of passage for every teen with a crooked smile. Invisalign® is a unique system of invisible aligners that help straighten teeth comfortably without metal bands, brackets or wires. The pieces are easily removable so you can eat, drink, brush and floss normally. Typically, the Invisalign® process takes about a year from start to finish. With this simple technique, there are no huge brackets darkening your smile, and you don't have to suffer through irritated lips or cheeks. Invisalign® can be used to eliminate crowding or large spaces between the teeth, overbites and underbites. However, Invisalign® only straightens your teeth, so if they are dark, discoloured or too short, additional treatment such as bonding or veneers will be needed to brighten up your smile. See www.invisalign.com.

Crowns and bridges

While porcelain veneers offer dazzling aesthetic results, they require adequate remaining tooth structure for their support. When there isn't adequate tooth structure, porcelain fused to metal crowns offers strength and durability. These restorations are stationary and are needed for teeth that have sustained significant structure damage, or to replace missing teeth.

Crowns and bridges may be placed on natural teeth or dental implants. A dental implant is an artificial tooth root that is placed into your jaw to hold a replacement tooth or bridge. Dental implants are an ideal option for people who have lost a tooth or teeth due to periodontal disease or an injury. Implants do not rely on neighbouring teeth for support and can look and feel completely natural. As a replacement for dentures, which often don't feel secure, implants can last you a lifetime.

Cosmetic contouring

A quick reshaping of your front teeth may be all you need to correct jagged, chipped or slightly uneven teeth. Crooked or asymmetrical teeth can be reshaped using a diamond drill, and a laser can be used to improve a gummy smile by raising the gum level. Porcelain laminates are made to sit on the tooth up to the newly raised gumline to eliminate a gummy smile.

SAVE YOUR SKIN (AND MAYBE YOUR LIFE TOO)

The incidence of skin cancer is growing at an alarming rate, making it the single most common form of cancer today. Sun exposure is universally cited as the primary cause of skin cancers because ultraviolet rays can damage DNA cells. Most cancerous lesions tend to be found on areas of the body that have been exposed to sunlight like the face, neck, arms, legs and chest. If detected and treated early, skin cancer has a cure rate of over 90 per cent.

Actually, life-threatening cancers can often be hidden under clothes. The most common location of skin cancer in women is the leg. It is also often found on the back where it can't be seen in the mirror.

Although fair-skinned people who sunburn easily are more prone to developing lesions, anyone can be at risk. A lifetime of summers at the beach covered in tanning oil with a SPF 6 can finally catch up with you. A 20-minute annual visit to your doctor or consultant dermatologist for a full body check from the top of your scalp to between your toes may actually save your life.

WARNING SIGNS

Look for spots that:
- change colour or get darker
- grow in size or thickness
- change in texture
- have an irregular shape
- are larger than the size of a pencil eraser
- don't heal
- scab, crust and itch
- are bleeding or oozing
- appear after age 21.

Skin cancer by definition is the uncontrollable growth of abnormal cells in a layer of the skin. It comes in many shapes, sizes and colours. **Actinic keratoses** – dry, crusty, flaky, often brown or pink, rough patches appear on the face, hands, lips or elsewhere. These lesions signal that the sun has damaged the skin, and are considered a precursor to skin cancer that one in six people will develop in their lifetime. They can show up even in young people. If left untreated, actinic keratoses can develop into any form of skin cancer.

Basal cell carcinoma – the most common form of skin cancer, this usually looks like raised, translucent lumps or growths.

Squamous cell carcinoma – characterised by crusty or scaly reddish patches, these can spread to other areas of the body.

Malignant melanoma – the least common but most deadly form of skin cancer, this can look like a dark mole or blemish and ranges from brownish or black. It can spread through the bloodstream and the lymphatic system.

When skin cancers are detected early, there are more effective options for treatment and cure. The biopsy is usually the first step to determining the best form of treatment, depending on the size, location and type of skin cancer. Cancerous growths can be surgically removed and excised, scraped away with a sharp instrument, and treated with liquid nitrogen to freeze the tissue. Laser technology can also be used to vaporise cancerous tissue in the layers of the skin and reduce pre-cancerous lesions like actinic keratoses.

The technique known as Mohs micrographic surgery is used to treat about one quarter of all skin cancers. Mohs surgery offers patients the highest cure rate and sacrifices the least amount of surrounding healthy tissue. This extremely accurate technique is performed under local anaesthetic. The tissue is flattened, frozen and divided into horizontal sections to check for the presence of a tumour. Repeated thin slices or layers of diseased tissue are taken until the margins of the lesion are clear and all the cancer has been safely removed.

Bits and Pieces

Ask The Beauty Junkie®

I have constant red marks on my face that are like acne, but not. Is there a laser that can help?

Rosacea is most common in fair- and thin-skinned individuals of northern European descent. It is a vascular condition and the redness and flare-ups can be controlled through medications, lifestyle changes and treatments. Avoid spices, curry, alcoholic beverages, steam, heavily fragranced skincare products, smoking and sun exposure. Your doctor may prescribe topical antibiotics to help prevent flushing and blushing. Intense pulsed light or fotofacial treatments can also be useful in keeping redness at bay. You will need a series of treatments, and after each session there should be a marked decrease in visible capillaries. See www.rosacea.org

Can anything get rid of melasma?

Melasma (also called the mask of pregnancy) usually shows up as dark patches on the cheeks and forehead, and around the mouth. These discolourations can sometimes look like a smudge, reminiscent of Ash Wednesday. The causes can be hormonal and genetic, and sun exposure brings it out. If you are taking birth control pills, ask your doctor if this may be the culprit. If you are prone to it, melasma may come up during pregnancy and the menopause. A series of glycolic or trichloracetic acid peels can blend your skin. Fraxel® laser also works well for melasma. Sun avoidance is mandatory to maintain skin lightening.

What works best to remove a tattoo?

A tattoo is one of those spur-of-the-moment things you tend to regret when you see your first grey hair – unless you're a rocker or a biker babe. Tattoos are not so easy to get rid of. Having a tattoo removed is much more expensive than getting one. Tattoo artists use heavy metals in their inks that can be resistant to many laser technologies; for example, black has iron, blue has cobalt. The age of the tattoo and the ink used affect how easy it is to obliterate – or not. The most commonly used lasers fall under the Q-switch

Plastic Makes Perfect

category because of the short, high-energy pulses of light used. Multiple sessions are needed to fade a tattoo out, and it may not go away completely.

Do facials make you look younger?

Facials should be a lovely, therapeutic and thoroughly relaxing experience. However, the primary goal of a 'facial' is not necessarily to make you look younger; most facials offer deep cleansing and hydration. They can moisturise and reduce impurities, as well as unclog pores and repair dry, stressed skin. The best facial for you should be based on your skin type and what you want to achieve. If you have severe acne, cysts, rosacea or broken capillaries, a facial may not be the ideal treatment for your skin. Facials can make spots worse, and squeezing or manipulating skin can spread bacteria. Steam can also cause veins to dilate and increase redness. A skilled beauty therapist or medical aesthetician can customise a treatment for your needs after conducting a thorough skin examination and taking a medical history.

Can using a scrub at home thin the skin?

A scrub exfoliates the skin to remove dead surface cells and leaves it feeling smoother. However, if a too-abrasive product is rubbed vigorously or too frequently, it can be irritating. Even sensitive skins need gentle exfoliation, just not as often as thicker, oily or younger skin types. If your skin is flushed, irritated, very sensitive or blotchy, don't scrub the skin until the skin's barrier returns to normal. Choose products that are mild and contain tiny particles or beads that are more gentle on the skin. If you have bought a scrub that is too abrasive for your face, try using it on your chest, arms or body skin instead. Never use a scrub around the eyes, on broken skin or right after waxing or using a depilatory.

Part IV

HOPE IN A JAR, TUBE, POT OR BOTTLE: LOTIONS AND POTIONS THAT MAKE A DIFFERENCE

12

Crèmes de la Creme: What Works

A re you a tried-and-true beauty junkie? If your bathroom shelves are overflowing with jars, bottles and tubes, you're not alone. Most women buy over three times more cosmetics than they could ever use in a lifetime. It's a bit like shoes – you never seem to have too many. We tend to have a short attention span for our skincare; we use it twice and forget about it. We all want instant effects and aren't willing to put the time into a product or regime to really give it a fair go.

SEVEN DEADLY SKIN SINS

- smoking
- sun exposure
- drinking alcohol
- being a couch potato
- overeating
- picking spots
- using the wrong products

When I do a consultation with a new client, I always put off any discussions about skin programmes and products until the end. There is never enough time to go through everything thoroughly when it comes to a chat about cosmetics. It's a girl thing – women have an insatiable appetite for talking about beauty products. Likewise here, I have saved the best for last.

AN OUNCE OF PREVENTION

The big question when faced with a weekend jaunt to Marbella is how much SPF is enough? An SPF measures only the amount of time it will take for you to get red. An SPF 15 is great for daily sun exposure, while an SPF 30 should be used during outdoor activities. The fairer your skin, or the more time you spend outside, the higher the SPF you should use.

Research suggests that the second day of sun exposure requires a higher SPF and more frequent application, and that a second application of sunscreen should be applied within 30 minutes of the first one to make up for areas you may have missed on the first go. Reapplication is considered essential, especially after sweating, swimming or towelling.

Although applying heavy-duty sunscreen and covering up with a T-shirt seems simple enough, sun protection doesn't begin and end with piling on creams. Covering up by wearing clothes should be part of the plan, and a gauzy little tank top won't pass muster. There is an entire industry devoted to producing protective garments from hats to trousers that are lightweight, comfy and surprisingly chic. Fabrics that have UPF (ultraviolet protection factor) ratings provide excellent skin coverage. For example, Coolibar (www.coolibar.com) labels its garments by how much protection they offer – for instance, 'Blocks 98 per cent UV' 'Excellent UV Protection', 'UPF 50+'. There are other considerations, such as the fact that less ultraviolet (UV) radiation passes through tightly woven or knitted fabrics. The smaller the spacing between the individual fibre strands of a fabric, the higher protection you will get. Darker colours of the same fabric type will usually absorb UV rays more than lighter shades. Many fabrics offer less UV ray protection when wet because UV rays pass through water better than through air. Most fabrics will get less protective as they age, so your old, faded polo shirts will be less effective in shielding you from the sun than this season's crisp Lacoste®.

Another hot tip is to add SunGuard® (see www.sunguardsunprotection.com) to your laundry, which can give your clothes a UPF of 30 with one cycle in your washing machine. The active ingredient is TINOSORB® FD, one of a new crop of UVA filters that is also used in sunscreens. It ensures that your clothes will absorb UV light rather than allow it to pass through the fabric to your body.

The usual recommendation when it comes to hats is a brim of at least three inches wide, which is especially good for protecting noses and ears. Philip Treacy meets Ascot usually won't do the job. Straw hats, Burberry visors, Texas-size Stetsons and baseball caps are also not very useful. For a hat to be truly protective, it should be cool and durable so that you'll keep it on, and made of or lined with treated material.

The same rules apply when it comes to sunglasses. All sunglasses will filter UV rays to some degree. Fashionista tints of pink, blue or purple may look good but they are poor light blockers. The lens should be uniform, not streaked or with dark or light spots. For very bright conditions, for instance when playing outdoor sports or boating, darker shades are better than tinted ones. Wrap-around frames with wide sides provide the best UV protection, and can also save you a fortune in Botox® by helping forestall crow's feet.

Another way to get your daily dose of UV protection is in a pill. Heliocare® Oral (see www.heliocare.co.nz) is a supplement containing antioxidants, green tea, beta-carotene and a natural fern extract. Taken daily, it is touted to minimise the damage caused by free radicals by corralling them before they can wreak havoc on your cells. This does not mean that taking one little capsule gives you the freedom to bake; rather it is an extra layer of protection.

UV rays are everywhere, even on a cloudy day in Gloucestershire. In fact, up to 80 per cent of the sun's rays can penetrate light clouds, mist and fog. Water, sand, snow and concrete can also reflect up to 80 per cent of the sun's damaging rays. UV levels are largely determined by latitude, cloud cover, time of year and time of day,

and they change every day. The closer you are to the equator, the higher the UV index (UVI). Thus you are less likely to go scarlet in northern Scotland than you would in southern France, but you can still get sun damage. The Met Office (www.metoffice.com) keeps track of the UVI for the UK and maintains links to websites that can give you the UVI for wherever you are going. UVI levels range from low (1–2) to extreme (11+). Generally, when the UVI forecast for the day is three to seven, you should seek shade during peak hours because photo damage and sunburn can occur and the risk of skin cancer increases. If it goes to eight or higher, stay inside.

CHANGING YOUR SKIN

A slapdash approach to skincare will fail miserably. Get serious about looking after your skin, or else you are wasting your time. It's like starting an exercise programme – working out once won't do the trick.

Just about any skin problem – sun damage, uneven skin tone, acne and blemishes or rosacea – can be improved by conscientious care and a daily ritual using a combination of ingredients. Sticking with the same old products as your skin changes won't work. Don't be afraid to experiment when your skincare stops working for you. And don't use the same tired old moisturiser that your mother used either. You don't have the same skin as your mother did then or now, and you need something that works for you.

If you are confused by the vast array of over-the-counter products and cosmeceuticals available, you're not alone. There's nothing worse than a skincare routine with a dozen steps. No one has the time any more for layering cream after cream. Keep it simple. Most women tend to pick and choose skincare without really understanding what will work best for their skin. While consultant dermatologists and skin experts can help, most people don't have access to them all the time, so get educated.

DO CREAMS REALLY WORK?

I get asked this question at least ten times a day. Creams absolutely work, but in a limited capacity. They can only get you so far. The main reason women are dissatisfied with their skincare is that their expectations are off the charts to begin with. Don't be dazzled by claims that sound miraculous – there is no facelift in a jar or filler in a bottle or toxin in a tube. Most cosmetic products use a relatively smaller concentration of the effective ingredients so that skin irritations are minimised. But that means the effectiveness may also be lessened. Many companies make great products, but they won't do much if your skin is in need of something more aggressive. Skincare is the place to start, in order to lay a foun-

Plastic Makes Perfect

dation for your beauty future, but eventually, over-the-counter products won't be enough. That's when it's time to move from cream to needle.

Prevention is usually easier and less painful than cure. If we knew then what we know now, we would have taken better care of our skin while we were young. Unfortunately, prevention is difficult to sell, especially to 25-year-olds with perfect, creamy complexions. While we are now seeing an increased use of sunscreens by younger people, sunscreens are not enough to prevent and protect skin from environmental ageing. It is difficult to demonstrate the preventive ageing effects of skincare. The only way to convince people is with compelling evidence that shows that prevention actually does reduce ageing.

THE SCIENCE BEHIND SKIN CREAMS

THE CREAM THAT ROCKED THE WORLD

You would have to be living under a rock not to have heard about Boots® Protect and Perfect Serum. This innocuous little bottle may actually set an all-time record as the most highly sought after skin care product in recent history. In a nutshell, this is a fairly generic antioxidant and retinol-based serum; better than some, and not as appealing as others. It is NOT, however, a facelift in a jar. Sorry to burst your bubbles, ladies....
www.boots.co.uk

'Clinically proven' – these two little words on a label invoke images of Petri dishes and microscopes. Behind the claims of scientific evidence, consumers expect some degree of rigour in ensuring that skincare products actually deliver the benefits they claim. But a clinical trial can be ten people using a product for a week and self-reporting their observations or a large-scale placebo-controlled study lasting several years under rigorously monitored conditions. Loose methodology or exaggerating average results

Crème de la Crème: What Works

273

compromises a skincare marketer's credibility. Clinical trials cost big bucks, and smaller brands just do not have the resources to do big studies for every product they launch. In general, the larger and longer the trial, the more likely the findings are to be accurate. All we can expect is for a brand to stand behind its science and make claims that can be substantiated. At the end of the day, the real proof in skincare is still every woman's standby, trial and error – and that has worked for centuries.

STRETCHING YOUR SKINCARE BUDGET

I am the original high-maintenance woman and the quintessential beauty product junkie. Although I am as drawn to deluxe packaging and sinfully delicious fragrances as the next woman, I have long recognised that when it comes to skincare there is absolutely no correlation between price and effectiveness. (One look in my make-up bag would confirm that I mix and match brands and price points, and get my cosmetics from all sorts of places including Selfridges, Sephora, Superdrug and even Safeway.)

One way to cut down on what you spend is to use less. We are programmed to pile on the creams to prevent wrinkles. But the truth is that women tend to overmoisturise. If your skin is dry and tight, moisturise it. If you want less moisture, use a lotion. If you want more, use a cream. If your skin is oily, use a lighter lotion or gel.

You don't have to take out a second mortgage to have great skin anymore. You can splurge on a few key treatment products and still save money if you are careful. But don't cut corners on all your skincare formulas. Buying cheaper products can sometimes mean sacrificing main ingredients that your skin craves. Lesser-quality products sometimes contain more water, so you need more to get the job done, and there go your savings.

Good-quality skincare products are very concentrated, so using a small amount (about the size of a pea) is often enough and can make them last longer. If you figure out the price of one ounce of an eye cream that costs £50 over three months, it comes to only pennies per day.

- If you have acne or blemishes, you should make treating them your top priority. It is worth spending more on medical products in order to maintain clearer skin.
- Splurge on a few great products you can't live without in the anti-ageing and treatment categories – for example, your favourite eye cream.
- Choose products that feel good texturally, wear well and you will enjoy using. If you don't like using a product, you won't apply it consistently enough to reap the real rewards, no matter what you paid for it.
- A daytime moisturiser with SPF can double up as your sun protection for overcast or indoor days. Clinique City Block has a range of good choices for under make-up.
- Spend more of your budget on your face than on your body. Fill in with less expensive cleansers, body scrubs and lotions, and hand creams.
- Sun care is one category where many pharmacy or mass brands are excellent. For city life, look for one that falls under the category of high (SPF 20–30) from a big company that has the funding to do serious research (Olay, L'Oréal, Soltan). For sports, go for extra high (SPF 30+), such as Uvistat Sun Cream SPF 50. At a pinch, you could use your children's sunscreen too.
- Watch expiration dates. The newer the product, the fresher the ingredients and the more effective it will be. Buy small sizes so that the shelf life does not expire before you get to the bottom of the jar.
- Learn which ingredients are the best fit for your skin concern, and seek out formulas that contain hot technologies at competitive prices. For example, if your skin craves minerals such as calcium for resiliency, try L'Oréal Age Perfect Pro Calcium Moist Pot for £14.99 before going for pricier versions.
- Gradual tan moisturisers come in all price ranges, and you need a

lot of any formula to see results. This is a good place to cut corners with drugstore brands.

- With premium brands, use a tester at the counter before investing in a product that isn't right for you. And when you make a purchase, always ask for samples of something else you are dying to try.
- If the product causes you to react or break out, ask for a refund or exchange it for something else. The return policy may be quite liberal in big stores (30–60 days), which gives you a chance to see results or not.
- Those foil packets found inside glossy magazines can come in really handy as a way to try out new products before buying.
- You don't have to spend a fortune on a good cleanser to get your skin clean and remove make-up. Look for multi-tasking products. One-step pharmacy wipes (Boots No. 7, Olay Daily Facials) do it all – cleanse, tone, remove face and eye make-up, and refresh. If they dry out, just add water to remoisten.
- Recycle skincare mistakes. If you bought something that doesn't work for you, pass it on to a friend or your mum instead of just throwing it in a drawer. If it makes you break out because it's too thick, use it on your hands, elbows and feet.
- Once you commit to a product, follow the directions and use it consistently for at least six weeks to really judge the benefits fairly.
- If you are on a tight budget, set an amount that you can comfortably spend, and start small. Add one key product at a time.
- Before you hit the high street, ask yourself what you want to tackle. Is it wrinkles? Brown spots? Dullness? Breakouts? Prioritise to avoid making mistakes and going over your budget.

WHAT WORKS – ANTI-AGEING

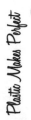

Women over 40 tend to visit their dermatologists more frequently to address common signs of ageing – dull, pale, tired skin that is less vibrant than the skin they had in their twenties. Skin care is the first step in beauty maintenance, so before you go under the knife, work with what you have. We can slow down the ageing process by seeking surgery alternatives that may work up to a point. Money is no object, but they must perform. Even drugstore brands are making very sophisticated claims now.

I am totally brand-agnostic. Just as I don't represent any doctors or clinics, I am also not a spokesperson for any skincare or cosmetic brand; nor do I have (or want) my name on the label. So these picks are based purely on what I like, what works for my clients and what I think has been tried and tested.

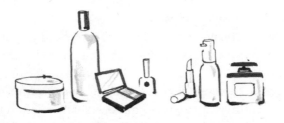

ANTI-AGEING SKINCARE ALL STARS

★ good value for money
★ ★ worth the spend
★ ★ ★ gotta have it

Face and neck (don't forget your décolleté too)

★ ★ ★ **SkinMedica™ TNS Recovery Complex®** A staple in America among gals in the know and the dermatologist's favourite, this unique formula contains human growth factors to fight skin ageing. See www.skinbrands.co.uk.

★ ★ ★ **Elizabeth Arden Prevage Anti-Aging Treatment** Through a partnership with Allergan (the Botox® people), this antioxidant formula contains idebenone to protect and restore skin. Also available especially for eyes, Prevage Eye Anti-Aging Moisturising Treatment. See www.elizabetharden.com.

★ ★ ★ **SkinCeuticals CEFerulic Acid** Serum containing 15 per cent pure L-ascorbic acid (vitamin C) and 1 per cent alpha tocopherol (vitamin E), with ferulic acid for maximum antioxidant potency. See www.skinceuticals.co.uk.

★ ★ **DDF® Dramatic Radiance TRF Cream™** Light firming lotion for the woman who doesn't like heavy moisturisers; replenishes skin with yeast and polysaccharides. See www.ddfskin.com.

★ ★ **N.V. Perricone MD Neuropeptide Facial Contour** The poor man's version of Perricone's signature Neuropeptide Facial Conformer, which has become a cult favourite among celebs for instant firming. See www.nvperriconemd.com.

★ ★ **NIA24™ Skin Strengthening Complex** Niacin-based repair cream for ageing skin. See www.nia24.com.

★ ★ **Zelens Night Cream** One of my clients sent me this duo of creams for day- and night-time use, and it is very rejuvenating. See www.zelens.co.uk

★ ★ **SeSha Skin Therapy Clinical Advanced Antioxidant Cream** Fully loaded moisturising cream with key antioxidants for skin renewal. See www.seshaskin.com.

★ ★ **Remergent DNA Repair Formula** A serum developed by a noted molecular biologist to encourage skin repair. See www.remergent-skin.com.

★ ★ **Freeze 24-7 Anti-Wrinkle Cream** Skin-plumping, wrinkle-releasing formula. See www.freeze247.com.

★ **Olay Regenerist Daily Regenerating Serum** This whole peptide-based range started a revolution of drugstore brands entering the cosmeceutical market, and remains a popular bargain-priced wrinkle reliever. See www.boots.co.uk.

Delicate eyelids

★ ★ ★ **DDF® Biomolecular Firming Eye Serum™** Featherweight serum for under eyes with proteins and peptides; great post-Botox®. See www.ddfskin.com.

★ ★ ★ **Estée Lauder Advanced Night Repair Eye Recovery Complex** Falls between a serum and a gel, to reduce puffiness and retexturise crêpiness. (My secret is to keep one in the fridge.) Try the restorative treatment, Estée Lauder Advanced Night Repair Concentrate Recovery Boosting Treatment, for weathered, damaged skin. See www.estéelauder.co.uk.

★ ★ ★ **Revision SkinCare Teamine Eye Complex** For dark circles and puffiness, a favourite in cosmetic surgery clinics. See www.revision-skincare.com.

★ ★ **Sisley Lip and Eye Contour Cream** Delicious anti-ageing treat for your skin. See www.sisley-cosmetics.com

★ **Talika Eye Decompress** Nifty single-use tablets that are immersed in blue liquid to form a soothing eye mask, perfect for jet lag and the morning after. See www.spacenk.com.

Body and hands

★ ★ ★ **SkinMedica™ Ceratopic® Replenishing Lotion** A miracle worker to speed up the recovery of extremely dry, cracked winterised skin. Perfect for hands, feet, elbows and knees. See www.skinbrands.co.uk.

★ ★ **Murad Firm & Tone Serum** Dimple-busting body beautifier. See www.murad.com.

★ ★ **MD Skincare Alpha Beta® Daily Body Peel** Skincare doesn't stop at your neck – your body needs exfoliation too. See www.mdskincare.com.

★ **AmLactin® 12 per cent Moisturising Cream** The ideal solution for rough, dry skin and winter itch, with 12 per cent lactic acid from the alpha hydroxy acid family. See www.upsher-smith.com.

★ **Clarins Super Restorative Redefining Body Cream** Caffeine-based slimming cream that leaves skin smooth. See www.clarins.co.uk.

FEAR OF FOUNDATION

Not wearing make-up or using it incorrectly can instantly add years to your face. Many women use the same old products for donkey's years, even though these may not be the best choices.

The ideal way to minimise imperfections lies in improving your skin as the first step. When your skin is clear and radiant, you have the ultimate foundation. Applying make-up on good skin is a real pleasure. The two go hand in hand – great skin and clever make-up. You can't really have one without the other. Bad skin and good make-up is just like putting a tiny plaster on a big wound – you can never cover it up sufficiently.

I am a woman who looks after her skin. My life is at my laptop in my office or hotels 24/7, and I rarely see the natural light of day. I use all sorts of creams and home treatments, and pop in for lasers and peels a few times a year. Fortunately, I got good skin genes. My mother and her mother before her had a creamy complexion even at an advanced age. (Don't be jealous – I got bad leg genes, so it's a wash!) Yet, even after these advantages, there is a sharp contrast between my face with make-up and without it.

For women over 35, make-up takes on a new art form. To soften lines you have to be meticulous about blending your foundation. Adjust the level of coverage for specific regions of your face, and remove any excess with a clean sponge. Avoid using greasy creams where you have the most lines. Foundation primers are usually silicone-based and can clog pores. Beware: anything slippery will make foundation migrate and sink into creases. If you have dry skin, choose a lighter texture with added hydrating ingredients. If you have oilier skin, stick with a matt formula to minimise shine.

No matter how flawless your complexion, a face with the right foundation will always look smoother, and have a more even tone with less redness and blotchiness. When you get the right foundation, and learn how to use it properly, you will see the difference it makes in your overall look. You don't absolutely have to wear foundation every day if you live in the country and spend your days riding horses. But as a grown up, you should at least know how to dress up your complexion when you want to put your best face forward.

FIVE POOR EXCUSES FOR NOT WEARING FOUNDATION AND SOME SOLUTIONS

Foundation washes me out Use a formula in a slightly darker shade to add some pigment and warm you up, and blend around jawline and hairline.

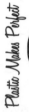

Make-up makes me break out Switch to an oil-free product that won't cause blemishes or clog pores.

It feels too heavy on my skin Try a tinted moisturiser or mineral-based brand that is super light, or use less of what you have.

The colour never looks right Choose your shade in natural daylight, or get an exact match that is custom blended and hand mixed just for you at a Prescriptives counter.

It doesn't stay on my skin Go with a matt formula that stays put and use powder to set all day.

Think of foundation as treatment, not just colour make-up. The best foundation looks and feels invisible on your skin. For me, no amount of money is too much to pay for a formula that really suits my skin and elicits compliments on how good it looks, even from total strangers.

GOOD FOUNDATIONS

Pick your budget, favourite type of coverage and finish, calculate your skin type and you've got it!

E = extra coverage for any time skin needs help
D = medium coverage for dry, dehydrated skin with wrinkles
M = matt finish for oily, shine-prone skin
L = light, for non-foundation wearers

Luxe (£60 and up)

D **La Prairie Cellular Radiance Lifting Foundation** Simply to die for. Gives your skin a soft, glowy and smooth finish. See www.laprairie.com.

E **La Prairie Skin Caviar Concealer Foundation** Comes with a creamy concealer in the silver cap. This works well when you need full coverage. See www.laprairie.com.

L **SK-II Airtouch Foundation** Light as a whisper, this stunning crimson

Crème de la Crème: What Works

compact offers a super-fine misting of sheer coverage. See www.sk2.co.uk.

D Estée Lauder Re-Nutriv Ultimate Lifting Creme Makeup SPF 15 Medium coverage, increased hydration, with SPF 15. See www.estée-lauder.co.uk.

M Sisley Botanical Makeup with Cucumber Mattifying treatment in a tube for oilier skin. See www.sisley-cosmetics.com.

Premium (£26–59)

D Chanel Vitalumiere Skin radiance is yours with this fluffy, creamy formula, in a medium wearable texture. See www.chanel.co.uk.

L La Mer The Treatment Fluid Foundation SPF 15 Light-reflecting for sheer coverage; perfect for younger skin and skin that is in good shape. See www.lamer.com.

D Bobbi Brown Luminous Moisturising Foundation One of her best-sellers, this medium-coverage liquid treatment is good for most skin types. See www.bobbibrown.com.

L Lancôme Aqua Fusion Teinté Sheer hydrating cream with SPF 15 and natural-looking tint. See www.lancome.co.uk.

E Kevyn Aucoin The Sensual Skin Enhancer Foundation Medium to full coverage in a pot; doubles as concealer. See www.kevinaucoin.com.

L By Terry Light-Expert To die for magic wand of feathery light colour to brush on all your imperfections for a flawless look. See www.byterry.com

M Glo Minerals™ Glo Camouflage Nice coverage from this range of mineral-based foundations, base and concealers. See www.glominerals.com

Cheap and cheerful (up to £25)

M Clarins Truly Matte Foundation A long-wearing shine-stopper. See www.clarins.co.uk.

L Lancôme Magic Matte Air-light Matte Mousse Foundation 12-hour medium coverage. See www.lancome.co.uk.

L Bourjois Happy Light Tinted Moisturising Foundation SPF 15 Oil-free sheer coverage for daywear. See www.bourjois.com.

M Clinique Clarifying Powder Makeup Oil-control and pore-minimising for thick, oily, blemish-prone skin. See www.clinique.co.uk.

D Mac Select SPF 15 Moistureblend Creamy compact; also comes in a liquid formula; with a natural finish, in dark shades too. See www.maccosmetics.com.

M Molton Brown Natural Skin Finish Shine-reducing powder to carry along all day. See www.moltonbrown.com.

IMMACULATE DECEPTION

If you use the wrong concealer to cover up brown spots, scars, dark circles, bruises and other post-surgery imperfections, you can unwittingly draw more attention to the area.

What not to do

- Use concealer on an oozing wound before your doctor gives you clearance.
- Apply creams or fragrance over suture lines.
- Wear make-up before it's an absolute must because you are going to be seen.
- Forget to remove all your camouflage make-up at bedtime.
- Abuse your newly lifted face or eyes by pulling and tugging to put on concealer.
- Wait until the morning you want to go out to hunt for camouflage make-up instead of having it on hand before you need it.
- Use your fingers instead of a clean sponge. (Avoid spreading bacteria.)
- Use latex sponges if you are sensitive or allergic to latex. Even the slightest contact with a latex sponge can make you flare up.
- Pile on opaque concealer so that it looks caked on – a little of a highly concentrated formula goes a long way.

Think of camouflage after surgery, injections or lasers as a layering process. Try full-coverage densely pigmented formulas that come in a pot, stick or tube. Liquids and creams are not usually opaque enough. If the cream is thick or firm, you can warm it up on your forehand or in the microwave for a few seconds. Green toners neutralise redness. Flat marks, scars and bruises will be easier to conceal than raised or depressed areas.

1. Choose a shade that best matches your skin tone. If you can't find an exact match, use a slightly lighter shade and blend over it with a liquid or cream foundation to normalise the colour.

NIP TIP
Don't be afraid to ask for help. Buy your foundation and concealer at a counter to get a good colour match. If you are trauma-tised about make-up, invest in a lesson with a professional make-up artist who can tailor a quick and simple routine that works for your skin and fits your lifestyle.

2. Start with clean, dry skin. Coat the edge of a sponge with a generous amount of concealer by swirling it around for a few seconds. Lightly pat (don't rub) the coated portion of the sponge on and around the outside of the area until you can no longer see the offending mark. Blend edges to avoid lines of demarcation.

3. Apply the rest of your make-up, avoiding the newly camouflaged area. If your concealer is off-colour, gently pat foundation over it until the colour blends nicely with the rest of your face.

4. Lastly, apply powder to absorb residual oils and pre-vent melting. Pressed translucent powder is less messy than loose. Or use a blush or powder brush and dust lightly over the camouflaged area. Repeat until the area is no longer shiny, and you're good to go.

5. Keep a powder compact with you to touch up any shine that comes on over the course of the day. Avoid conscious and subconscious face touch-ing, which can wipe away your brilliant camouflage job. Leave it alone and forget about it.

Great camouflage products to cover up all your flaws (not that you have any . . .).

About face

Extra-strength cover-ups for post surgery, injections, laser or just natural ageing and sun damage.

Bobbi Brown Creamy Concealer Kit Comes in eight shades for an easy colour match. Use with the Dual Ended Concealer Corrector Brush. See www.bobbibrown.com.

Prescriptives Flawless Skin Concealer Thirty shades with SPF 27. See www.prescriptives.com.

Amazing Cosmetics Amazing Concealer Comes in a tube, so it is easy to blend and lasts forever; a potent secret of make-up artists that is a winner. See www.amazingcosmetics.com.

Estee Lauder DoubleWear Stay in Place Concealer SPF 10 Easy to use to cover flaws and spots and stays where you put it. www.esteelauder.co.uk.

Cover FX Total Coverage Cream Foundation Opaque yet gentle enough for sensitive skin; 40 shades. See www.coverfx.com.

Dermacia® MD Lycogel Full coverage for post-laser and lifts with SPF 30. See www.dermaciamd.com.

Under eyes

For dark circles, hollows and raccoon eyes, gently place or pat concealer on and don't rub.

Jane Iredale Active Light™ Brush-on formula that conceals without dulling and minimises dark circles with vitamin K. See www.janeiredale.com.

Clinique All About Eyes Ideal solution for dark circles that stays in place for hours. See www.clinique.co.uk.

By Terry Multicare Concealer Silky elegant texture for under eyes to carry in your bag. See www.byterry.com.

L'Oreal Infallible Concealer High-coverage stick formula. See www.boots.co.uk.

Body under cover

To cover up veins, scars, age spots or post-laser marks, start with body moisturiser and then apply make-up.

CoverBlend by Exuviance Corrective Leg and Body Makeup SPF 18 Opaque coverage with titanium dioxide for broad-spectrum sun protection. See www.neostrata.com.

Coverderm Perfect Legs SPF 16 Creamy cover-up for veins and bruises www.coverderm.com

YOUR SEARCH FOR SMOOTHER SKIN

Getting clinical skincare results at home is a bonus – especially for working mums and managing directors who haven't got the time to pop in for treatments in between meetings. These days you can make your skin glowing and young-looking in the privacy of your own bathroom. Exfoliation is a key part of every skincare regime. Physical exfoliants (face brushes, pads, scrubs loaded with sugar, salt, polyethylene beads) work by sloughing away dead or excess cells that clog pores and cause dullness. Chemical exfoliants include peeling solutions and topical products. Both gentle chemical and physical exfoliation work well, and you can switch off as needed.

DIY must-haves

Lancôme Resurface Peel Resurfacing and Soothing System Brilliant for even the clumsiest peelers, this system leaves you smooth as a baby's bum in about five minutes. Try **Resurface Microdermabrasion**

Body too. See www.lancome.co.uk.

DDF 5 per cent Daily Cleansing Pads Mild enough to use daily, or twice daily during summer or on oily skin. DDF makes the softest, most user-friendly pads on the market. See www.ddfskin.com.

Dr Brandt Microdermabrasion Creamy skin polish with magnesium oxide crystals scrub to slough dead cells away. See www.drbrandtskincare.com.

Roc Renewex™ Microdermabrasion Expert System As good as expensive systems that work the same way, this handheld unit has a sponge applicator with an aluminum oxide cream to spin away dead cells and pore-clogging debris. See www.boots.co.uk.

Clarisonic® Cleansing Brush DIY super cleansing for dirty, gritty, city skin. See www.clarisonic.com.

L'Oréal Renoviste Anti-Ageing Glycolic Peel Kit Cheap and cheerful easy-to-use version. See www.boots.co.uk.

Dr Brandt Microdermabrasion in a Jar Creamy skin polish with magnesium oxide crystals scrub to slough dead cells away. See www.drbrandtskincare.com

Natura Bisse Glyco Extreme Peel Peptide-based peeling with beta hydroxy acid for gentle but effective exfoliation. See www.naturabisse.com

Agera Rx Microderma Crystal C System Lactic acid, peptide and Vitamin C combo to dissolve dead cells. See www.agerarx.co.uk.

DDF MesoInjection Healthy Cell Serum A novel product designed to mimic the effects of a mesolift in rejuvenating slack, dehydrated, ageing skin. See www.ddfskin.com.

THE POWER OF VITAMIN A

Retin-A®, containing vitamin A, is considered the mother of all cosmeceuticals. Vitamin A is the first vitamin to be used topically for the treatment of damaged skin. Today, the term 'vitamin A' is applied to retinol (vitamin A alcohol), retinal (vitamin A aldehyde) and tretinoin (vitamin A or retinoic acid). Vitamin A stimulates cell activity and the production of collagen, and helps to renew and exfoliate the skin. This makes it an ideal night-time treatment to restore the damage done to your skin during the day.

Retinoids, specifically Retinova® and Avage® (Tazorac®), are the only FDA-approved wrinkle creams. The biggest problem is that people don't stick with them because of the side-effects of dryness and redness. Retinol is retinyl alcohol, and gets naturally converted into retinoic acid in the skin. It improves fine lines, but doesn't do as much for pigment and wrinkle reduction as its stronger, older cousin Retin A does. Retinoic acid includes Retin-A®, Retinova®, Retin-A Micro® and other prescription-strength vitamin A derivatives.

Retinova® (Janssen-Cilag) contains the active ingredient tretinoin 0.05 per cent in an emollient cream, and is the first drug licensed for treating sun-damaged skin. For some unexplained reason, it has been discontinued in the UK, yet some independent chemists still carry a limited supply. (Scoring a vial of crack cocaine on the streets of east London would appear to be far easier than buying an innocent little tube of wrinkle cream from a legitimate chemist.) It is used once a day at bedtime, tapering off to three times per week. Using it more will not make it work any faster. The mineral oil base can be greasy for oily skin. Expect some flaking at first, and a daily broad-spectrum SPF is a must. Other retinoic acids in the UK include Retin-A® Cream (Tretinoin) and Differin® (Adapalene), which also require a prescription from your doctor. None of these should be used while pregnant or nursing.

What is the alternative?

Airol® Crème 0.05 per cent A Retin-A/Retinova® substitute from Pierre Fabre Pharma, available by prescription. See www.wigmore-medical.com.
Environ® Intensive Range Developed by a South African plastic surgeon, this progressive skincare range has three retinol strengths. Available at clinics only. See www.environ.co.za.
Skinceuticals Retinol 0.5 Night cream for cell renewal. See www.skinceuticals.co.uk.

WHAT DOES SUNSCREEN DO FOR YOU?

A broad spectrum sunscreen should be your 'go to' beauty product.

UVA rays are known as the ageing rays, whereas UVB rays are the burning rays. Many products are adequate to protect against UVB, but beware the dangers of UVA rays. The European Commission has ruled that all sunscreen products will have to state whether they offer low, medium, high or very high protection, and must not only give their Sun Protection Factor (SPF) rating for UVB rays but also show what protection they offer against UVA rays which are also responsible for deadly skin cancers. The word 'sunblock' has also been deemed to be misleading because it implies that you are fully protected, which is not always the case. I would rather have my clients buy a cheap and cheerful sun care product with good protection and layer it on generously, than splurge on an expensive brand that they might only use in small doses. Without sun protection, none of the anti-ageing treatments in this book are going to do you much good. And SPF 15 is a minimum – don't think that an SPF 8 is doing you much good.

GIVE YOUR SKIN THE ALL CLEAR

There is no doubt that coping with niggling skin problems gets harder as you get older. Sometimes acne goes away, but it can get worse, or spots can creep up on you even if you had clear skin as a teen. Wrinkles and blotches are a fact of life past the age of 30. Redness shows up from sun damage and skin thinning. Try these short-term solutions which can really help.

Spots and blemishes

Biore Ultra Deep Cleansing Pore Strips Still works for nasty blackheads around the nose. See www.boots.co.uk.

Murad Clarifying Cleanser Banish blemishes where they live. See www.murad.com.

Neutrogena Visibly Clear Deep Cleansing Wipes Easy to use wipes that take grime away and unclog pores. Good for younger, oily complexions. www.boots.co.uk.

Zeno® Pro Acne Clearing Device As slim and sleek as your mobile, this nifty device zaps pimples before they ruin your day. See www.myzenoeurope.com.

Blotches and patches

Olay® Definity Correcting Protective Lotion SPF 15 Helps mild skin discolourations; good for daytime use. See www.olay.com.

Agera Rx Phyto Lightening Cream Part of a range of clinical-strength skin lighteners formulated with mulberry, bearberry and kojic acid. See www.agerarx.co.uk.

Obagi® Nu-Derm Blender® From the master of hyperpigmentation solutions, this formula is intended for use with Retin-A® to promote even complexions. See www.obagi.com.

Amelan® Depigmentation Treatment (Cosmelan®) Two-step skin-bleaching system consisting of a mask and cream, containing a blend of active botanicals. See www.amelan.co.uk.

Flushing and blushing

Clinique Cx Antioxidant Rescue Serum Potent formula for minimisng skin's redness and flare-ups. See www.clinique.co.uk.

B. Kamins Booster Blue Rosacea Treatment Fragrance-free soother based on their patented maple compound. See www.bkamins.com.

DDF Redness Relief Controls flare-ups with active botanicals. See www.ddfskin.com.

Avene Diroseal Treatment Cream French pharmacist's secret for flushing skin. See www.boots.co.uk.

Cutanix® Dramatic Relief Safe, gentle anti-redness cream that works all day. See www.cutanix.com.

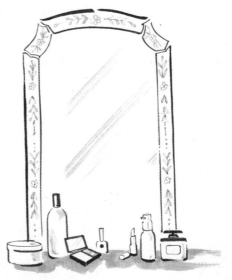

Ask The Beauty Junkie®

How can I tell if my skincare is working?
Use it as directed for at least six full weeks consistently to judge fairly. Get a second opinion; ask your partner or a girlfriend who will tell you the truth if they see an improvement. If you are not getting remarks like 'Your skin looks amazing!' it may not be getting the job done.

What helps to get rid of open or enlarged pores?
Pores are not really open, but there are several methods of making them look smaller and tighter. Keeping pores clean is a good place to start. Regular exfoliation transforms clogged and enlarged pores. When cell production speeds up, the epidermis becomes thicker. Since open pores are exposed to the air, the oil inside them becomes oxidised and turns black, which makes them more noticeable. Exfoliants such as glycolic acid, lactic acid and salicylic acid work by dissolving the bonds between cells on the top layer of the skin so that they shed more easily and evenly. Apply a mild alcohol-free toner after cleansing to close pores.

Microdermabrasion treatments are a good next step and intense pulsed light treatments keep pores looking taut and firm.

Will drinking more water make me look younger?
This is one of the greatest beauty myths since the beginning of time. How much water you drink has little to do with ageing, except perhaps if you have been trekking across the Sahara and look like a wrinkled prune from dehydration. There are many obvious health benefits of drinking water; however, if that is your number-one anti-ageing strategy, call for back-up or go to Plan B.

Do creams that claim to be better than Botox® do anything?
The power of peptides is being harnessed to mimic the effects of injectable botulinum toxin. Peptide creams can have a visible effect on your wrinkles, but they work in a totally different and much less potent way. No topical cream can penetrate deep into your mus-

cles with the precision of a needle. These products work on the lines and wrinkles, and not on the muscle directly as Botox® does.

What should I put on my face first?

If you are using an anti-ageing or anti-acne product, put the medicine on first; let your skin dry and then pat on sunscreen; and lastly, apply foundation. Don't rub each layer in as you apply, to avoid blending it all together. Otherwise, you can apply chemical sunblocks, such as Avobenzone, first. Chemical blockers bind to the skin and absorb UV light. Physical blockers reflect the energy back out into the environment, so these can go on last.

13

High Maintenance: Keeping Up Appearances

THE WHOLE IS GREATER THAN THE SUM OF ITS PARTS

Think of maintenance as what makes you not want to dive into the ladies room when you run into an ex during daylight. We can roll back the years with a combination of small treatments that really work.

There is no facelift in a jar. Great skin is not about looking 18 when you're 80. It's about choosing a sensible approach to caring for your skin, keeping it looking radiant and healthy, and making the most of what you have. It's the canvas that counts the most. You can have the most brilliant cosmetic surgeon in the world, but if you started out with wrinkled, leathered, damaged, thin skin, everything will be tighter but you will still have yellow and brown spots, lines, wrinkles and blotches.

The latest thinking is that the best results come from combining treatments. By mixing non-invasive procedures, a doctor can address multiple signs of ageing in one or two sessions. For example, the quartet of Botox®, chemical peel, laser toning and Restylane® filling is a winning combination that can dramatically rejuvenate the eye area. These treatments take literally minutes to do, and if you're not happy with the results, you're not committed. In about six months, your face will return to its former self. It's more like borrowing time.

Combination therapy is the buzzword of the day. It is rare for a woman to walk into her cosmetic surgeon's rooms with only one thing on her mind. Rather, she will come in with a laundry list of big and little things she wants corrected, improved, obliterated or enlarged from head to toe. And with a long list of new advances set to hit the market, the future of the rejuvenation category looks very bright.

THE FUTURE OF FLAWLESS

The Academy of Anti-Aging Medicine (www.worldhealth.net) suggests that by the year 2049, our maximum life expectancy will have reached 129. If you accept this premise, then you had better get cracking!

GROWING YOUR OWN CELLS

Stem cell science has the potential to revolutionise medicine. Embryonic stem cells are taken from an embryo, whereas adult stem cells are taken from a person or from the umbilical cord. In theory, stem cells can grow and develop into any spare part you need – for example, a new liver. Stem cells can be used to create the cells responsible for fighting diseases and putting those cells in the body. Research is currently under way for diabetes, Parkinson's disease, heart disease, breast cancer, Crohn's disease and many other diseases.

The prospects are very exciting. One day, cosmetic surgery may be obsolete as a way to erase wrinkles and fine lines or to create bigger breasts. Where a scalpel was once required, stem cell therapy could do the job. Although stem cell applications on the vanity market may have to wait, hair follicular stem cells, tooth stem cells and skin stem cells all show promise as ways to restore hair to a bald head, teeth to a toothless mouth and new skin to people with traumatic burn scars. A group from Japan reported on enriching liposuctioned fat with fat-derived stem cells and using the material successfully for breast enlargement. Stem cell research may one day allow breast cancer survivors to take advantage of natural replacement after a mastectomy. Unfortunately, the use of stem cells to regenerate tissue could still be a few decades away.

BALDNESS GENE

Common baldness doesn't happen without the presence of specific inherited genes. Until now we didn't know which genes were involved. Research scientists have discovered a gene that plays an important role in male hair loss on the X chromosome. Men inherit the X chromosome from their mothers, while women inherit an X from each parent. When it comes to going bald, men take after their maternal grandfather rather than their father, although it may be possible for this gene to be passed directly from father to son. The gene affects the androgen receptor, a protein that helps activate male hormones. However, baldness is not caused by just one little gene. Nevertheless, isolating the gene that contributes to hair loss is the first step in finding a cure to baldness. Genetic engineering to prevent baldness may be closer than you think.

A NEW FACE

In 2005, Isabelle Dinoire became the world's first partial face transplant patient. The procedure was performed in France by a team of surgeons in order to repair Isabelle's face after a dog attack. The doctors removed tissue from a donor's nose and mouth and used it to repair Isabelle's facial disfigurement.

In the past, ear and scalp transplants have been performed, but a face transplant is a recent advance that improves facial appearance after severe disfigurement from trauma. The concept is relatively straightforward, at least on paper. A face transplant involves healthy tissue being taken from a donor. Then the traumatised tissue is removed from the patient. The healthy tissue from the donor is then surgically attached to where the recipient needs it.

The technique is so new that standards for face transplant surgery have not yet been established. The medical community has conflicting opinions about face transplants, and there are concerns about how the

Plastic Makes Perfect

immune system will respond to foreign bodies. These issues require further research, but the prospects are pretty incredible.

THE KNIFE COACH® WISH LIST

If I could close my eyes and make a wish, this is what I hope to see in the near future.

More female cosmetic surgeons In the US, there are still very few women in plastic surgery, although there are many terrific women in dermatology and cosmetic dentistry. We need more women in the operating theatres.

Better methods to tighten sagging skin sans scars Just imagine doctors being able to shrink and firm up loose skin without any surgery. We are getting closer by the nanosecond . . .

A way to pulverise fat cells without surgery Even a few years ago, this would never have seemed possible, but today we are almost there, with new devices under development that can make us slimmer without scars.

Tanning pill Let's hope we see an end to tanning booths as we know them. The risk of skin cancer belittles the risk of premature wrinkling. DHA, or dihydroxyacetone, is the main ingredient in sunless tanners today and they work well. A true sun-free tanning drug will save lives.

Longer-lasting toxin Although I love my Botox®, I would love it better if I had to go back not every four to five months but rather six to nine months, or even longer.

Fast-healing scars This too seems as if it is almost a reality. The innovation of newly designed sutures for wound closure is making possible shorter scars that close large portions of tissue in a neater way.

Skincare based on your DNA Some day soon, someone is going to take the guesswork out of skincare by coming up with an effective way to harness the power of your own personal blueprint. Your DNA could predict if you're prone to wrinkles, and then determine what skincare products you need for your individual cells.

Skin cancer vaccine A vaccine treatment called Oncophage®, made from an individual person's tumours, is currently being investigated as an aid to the treatment of melanoma, the most deadly form of skin cancer.

DIY beautification As a practised multi-tasker, I would love to see more homecare devices for skin rejuvenation, teeth whitening, light-based hair removal, acne zappers, no-needle mesotherapy, and cellulite and fat busters. These are coming.

The scope of cosmetic medicine is expanding and is no longer being performed only with a scalpel. The future lies in integrating surgical and non-surgical procedures. With a little luck, when I update this book in a year or two, everything on my wish list will be old news.

Abdominoplasty Plastic surgery of the abdomen, or tummy tuck, in which excess fatty tissue and skin are removed.

Ablation Vaporisation of the most superficial layers of skin.

Acne An inflammatory eruption of the skin that occurs when a hair follicle gets plugged with sebum and dead cells.

Actinic keratosis A lesion that is dry, scaly, rough and tan or pink, caused by sun exposure and considered pre-cancerous.

Alar base The wing-like structures at the base of the nose.

Allergen A substance that can cause allergic reaction.

Alopecia A condition of hair loss.

Alpha hydroxy acid (AHA) A group of acids derived from foods such as fruit and milk, which can improve the texture of the skin by removing layers of dead cells.

Anatomic breast implant Teardrop-shaped implant (as opposed to the round style), designed to look more like a natural breast.

Antibiotic A drug that destroys bacteria or slows down its growth.

Antioxidant A substance that soaks up free radicals (such as vitamins C, E, A, grape seed and green tea). See also Free radicals.

Areola The pigmented skin around the nipple.

Arnica Botanical derived remedy from a mountain plant with antiseptic, astringent, antimicrobial and anti-inflammatory properties.

Autologous Occurring naturally in a certain type of tissue of the body.

Barbed sutures Sutures with barbs or cogs that can be attached to tissue to tighten the skin and close wounds more effectively.

Basal cell carcinoma Cancer of one of the innermost cells of the deeper epidermis of the skin.

Benign Non-cancerous.

Beta hydroxy acid See Salicylic acid.

Bleaching agents Substances that slow down or block the production of melanin to fade areas of hyperpigmentation (hydroquinone, kojic acid, azelaic acid).

Blepharoplasty (eyelid plasty) Surgery to remove excess fat, muscle and/or skin around the eyes.

Botox® See Botulinum toxin.

Botulinum toxin A toxin that is injected into muscles to temporarily reduce their activity and eliminate expression lines of the face and around the eyes and lines on the neck. Botox® is the trade name for this treatment.

Brachioplasty Surgery involving an incision in the armpit and continuing towards the inside of the elbow to remove excess skin and fat from the upper arms.

Broad-spectrum sunscreen Sunscreen that blocks the effects of UVA and UVB light. See also UVA light and UVB light.

Browlift See Forehead lift.

Buccal fat pads Fat pads located in the cheek, also known as the fat pad of Bichet.

Cannula Long, thin hollow tubular instrument used to extract fat during liposuction.

Capillary The smallest type of blood vessel in the body, commonly found on the face or legs.

Capsular contracture Scar tissue that forms in the pocket surrounding a breast implant and becomes hardened and distorted.

Carbon dioxide laser Laser technology that can be used to resurface moderate to deep facial wrinkles and scars. It can also be used as a cutting tool.

Cauterise To burn or sear abnormal tissue with a cautery such as a laser.

Cellulite Deposits of fat, toxins and fluids trapped in pockets beneath the skin.

Cheeklift See Mid-facelift.

Chemical peel Solution applied to specific areas to peel away the skin's top layers, such as alpha hydroxy acid, beta hydroxy acid or trichloroacetic acid (TCA).

Collagen Protein fibres in the skin's second layer that gives it resiliency, suppleness and tone, and breaks down with age.

Collagenase An enzyme that breaks down collagen.

Columella The strip of skin dividing the nostrils at the base of the nose.

Commissure The area where two anatomic parts meet, as in the corner of the eye or the lips; typically refers to a fold or crease.

Congenital defect Abnormality formed at birth.

Coronal Of or pertaining to the top of the head or skull.

Corrugator Muscle that is responsible for causing the glabellar (vertical) lines that form between the eyebrows.

Cosmeceutical Substance falling between the classification of a drug and a cosmetic, i.e. a non-prescription over-the-counter formulation that provides pharmaceutical benefits.

Craniofacial surgery Reconstructive surgery of the face and head.

Cross linked Refers to the bonds that link one polymer chain to another, as in fillers, which usually makes the substance thicker and of longer duration.

Crust Surface layer formed by the drying of a bodily secretion.

Cryosurgery Surgery in which diseased or abnormal tissue (such as a tumour or wart) is removed by freezing (for instance by the use of liquid nitrogen).

Cupid's bow The double curve of the upper lip that resembles a curved bow with reversed curve ends.

Cyst Large, solid bump formed within hair follicles, located deep within the skin.

Deflation A rupture or tear in the shell of a breast implant that causes the filler (saline, silicone gel or other) to leak out and the implant to flatten.

Dermabrasion Non-surgical resurfacing procedure in which a hand-held rotary wheel is used to remove the top layer of skin.

Dermatitis Inflammatory condition of the skin that is characterised by itching and redness.

Dermis Layer of skin composed of collagen and elastin, lying beneath the epidermis (outer layer) and above the subcutaneous layer.

Diode Contact laser technology that cuts and coagulates tissue.

Dry eye A condition of the eyelids that causes dryness, blurred vision

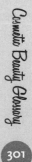

and the eyes to feel gritty.

Ecchymosis Bruising marked by a purple discolouration of the skin.

Ectropion A condition when the lower eyelid is pulled downwards as a result of loose eyelid skin or muscles or too much skin having been removed. Also called lid retraction.

Edema An excess accumulation of fluid in the connective tissue.

Elastin A protein similar to collagen that makes up elastic fibres.

Electrocautery The burning of tissue with an electric current by use of a specially designed apparatus.

Encapsulation The growth of a membrane around any part so as to enclose it in a capsule.

Endoscopic surgery Surgery performed using an endoscope, a small tube-like instrument equipped with fibre-optic lighting, introduced into the body through a tiny incision so that the surgeon can see the area on a video monitor while performing an operation (such as endoscopic browlift, breast augmentation or facelifting).

Epidermis The skin's outermost layer.

Epithelialisation Regeneration of the epithelium or superficial layer of the skin, as occurs after laser resurfacing.

Erbium: YAG A type of ablative laser that produces energy in a wavelength that penetrates the skin and is readily absorbed by water.

Erythema Redness of the skin, as in post laser or other resurfacing.

Excision Surgical removal.

Exfoliation The regular removal of dead skin cells from the epidermis.

Extrusion The erosion of skin that causes an implant (chin, lip, breast) to become partially exposed.

Eyelid plasty See Blepharoplasty.

Facelift See Rhytidectomy.

Fascia The sheet of connective tissue that covers the muscles, sometimes used as a graft material.

Fat embolus Globules of fat that can infiltrate the bloodstream during surgery, causing a mass that can result in serious complication and death.

Fibrin sealant A natural agent for the achievement of rapid hemostasis and tissue sealing; used instead of stitches or staples in surgery. Also called tissue glue.

Plastic Makes Perfect

Fibroblast A cell from which connective tissue develops.

Filler A category of substances that are either injected or implanted to shape and form overlying tissue.

Follicles See Pores.

Forehead lift Cosmetic surgery that pulls up droopy brows and upper lids, and improves wrinkling and vertical and horizontal frown lines. Also called a browlift.

Free radicals Destructive form of oxygen molecules generated by each cell in the body that destroy cellular membranes.

Frontalis The muscle that enables the brows to move up and down, and contributes to the formation of horizontal wrinkles of the forehead.

General anaesthetic Total anaesthesia and loss of consciousness so that you don't feel anything. A breathing tube is placed in the airway.

Genioplasty Cosmetic surgery to add projection to the chin. The bones are broken so that the chin area can be moved forward and secured in place.

Glabella The area between the eyebrows in the centre of the forehead where deep vertical lines and creases often develop.

Glycolic acid An effective exfoliant that renews skin by dissolving dead skin cells.

Graft A piece of tissue (such as fat, cartilage, bone, skin, etc) that is totally removed from one part of the body and transferred to another area of the body.

Growth factors Proteins that repair and preserve tissues and stimulate blood cell production.

Hair follicle The cylindrical site in the epidermis in which the hair shaft and sebaceous gland are located.

Hematoma A localised accumulation of blood in the skin caused by a blood vessel wall rupture – a possible complication of surgery that may have to be drained.

Hyaluronic acid An acid found naturally in the body that helps retain the skin's natural moisture.

Hyperpigmentation Increased pigment in the skin that may be caused by hormones, skin injury or sun exposure.

Hypertrophic scar Thickened, raised or red scar tissue.

Hypertrophy Enlarged or thickened organ or area of tissue.

Hypoallergenic A substance with a low chance of causing allergy or skin irritation.

Hypopigmentation Reduction in the pigment cells in the skin, resulting in skin lightening.

Inframammary crease The skin crease or fold that lies beneath the breast.

Intense pulsed light Very strong light without a light beam that is one wavelength (colour) or coherent.

Jaw Term used to describe the maxillae and mandible and soft tissue surrounding the bony structure.

Keloid Enlarged, permanent and thickened scar formations that are more common in darker skin types.

Lactic acid A component of the skin's natural moisturising factor.

Lateral hooding Excess fold of skin between the eyebrow and the outer portion of the upper eyelid.

Lentigines Condition caused by chronic sun exposure. Also known as freckles, liver spots, age spots or brown spots.

Lesion Any kind of wound growth or sore on the skin caused by injury or disease.

Lidocaine A local anaesthetic used topically on the skin and mucous membranes. Also called xylocaine.

Lipoplasty/liposuction A procedure in which localised collections of fat are removed from the face and/or body by using a high-vacuum device through small incisions.

Local anaesthetic Medications (usually in the 'caine' family) that are injected into a surgical or treatment site to cause temporary localised numbness.

Lumpectomy Surgery to remove a cancerous lesion and a small amount of surrounding tissue.

Lymphatic system A network of structures, including ducts and nodes, that carry lymph fluid from tissues to the bloodstream.

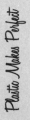

Melanoma The most deadly type of skin cancer, which spreads rapidly and is typically related to sun exposure.

Malar bags A pouch of loose skin and fluid that sometimes occurs with age below the lower eyelid area.

Malar fat pad A structure that sits in the second layer of the face below the cheekbone that is frequently repositioned during facial rejuvenation procedures.

Malarplasty Cosmetic surgery to achieve cheekbone reduction or augmentation.

Mammogram A special X-ray of the breast which detects lumps in breast tissue.

Mandible Jawbone.

Marionette lines The vertical creases that form in the corners of the mouth towards the jowls.

Mask of pregnancy See Melasma.

Mastectomy Surgical removal of the breast and/or some of the lymph nodes in the armpit.

Mastopexy Surgical breastlift procedure performed to re-shape the breast.

Melanin The pigment that gives skin its colour.

Melanocytes Cells that produce melanosomes, which in turn produce melanin.

Mentoplasty Surgery of the chin whereby its shape or size is altered.

Melasma (cholasma) Localised brown patches on the forehead, cheeks and upper lip caused by hormones and sun exposure. Also called the mask of pregnancy.

Mentalis A muscle that originates in the incisive fossa of the mandible, inserts in the skin of the chin, raises the chin and pushes up the lower lip.

Microdermabrasion An intensive treatment for deeply penetrating pore cleansing and skin-cell exfoliation.

Mid-facelift A surgical procedure designed to lift sagging areas in the mid-face, including around the cheekbone areas below the eyes. Also called a cheeklift.

Midline An imaginary vertical line that divides the face or body into two equal areas.

Milia Tiny skin cysts that resemble whiteheads.

Mitral valve prolapse Cardiopathy resulting from the mitral valve not regulating the flow of blood between the left atrium and left ventricle of the heart.

Musculature The system or arrangement of muscles in a body or a body part.

Nasion The depression at the root of the nose that indicates the junction where the forehead ends and the bridge of the nose begins.

Nasolabial folds The region of the face between the nose and the corners of the lip; commonly referred to as smile lines.

Non-ablative laser resurfacing A new class of laser treatment that does not produce a deep burn and is much less invasive than other laser treatments.

Orbicularis oculi The muscular body of the eyelid encircling the eye and comprising the palpebral, orbital and lacrimal muscles.

Orbit The cavity in the skull where the eyeballs, eye muscles, nerves and blood vessels rest.

Osteotomy The operation of dividing a bone or cutting a piece out of it.

Otoplasty Reparative or cosmetic surgery of the auricle of the ear.

Pectoralis The muscle that is located between the rib cage and the chest tissue.

Peptides A chain of various amino acids or proteins.

Periareolar The area around the areola.

pH The degree of acidity or alkalinity, for example in the solution of products.

Photo ageing Damage to the skin caused by cumulative exposure to the sun – i.e. wrinkles, age spots, fine lines.

Photosensitivity The skin's photosensitivity or sensitivity to light is such that chemicals or topical ingredients cause it to be reactive when exposed to sunlight, resulting in problems such as inflammation, hyperpigmentation and swelling.

Platysma A thin sheet of muscle located just beneath the skin of the chin and neck.

Platysmal band Vertical strands of the muscle of the neck.

Poly-L-lactic acid A biodegradable, non-allergenic dermal filler.

Pores Tiny holes or follicles that house fine hairs. Oil glands at the

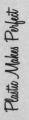

base of each follicle produce sebum, which travels up the hair shaft on to the surface of the skin to provide lubrication. Also called follicles.

Postinflammatory hyperpigmentation Pink-to-brown colour in the skin that occurs after a wound or pimple heals.

Procerus Muscle that works with the corrugator muscles and contributes to the vertical frown lines between the eyebrows.

Ptosis Pronounced 'toe-sis', a term for drooping, as in eyelids, breasts and brows.

Radio-frequency treatment A heat-energy treatment that penetrates deeply into the skin, shrinking both scars and oil glands. It may also tighten collagen.

Retin-A® (Tretinoin) A topical medication derived from vitamin A that is used to treat photo ageing and acne.

Retinol A gentler non-prescription-strength alternative to retinoic acid. Retinol is a fast, active form of vitamin A that works deep under the surface of the skin to visibly reduce lines and wrinkles.

Retinyl palmitate The reaction of retinol and palmitic acid, which normalises skin by significantly changing skin composition to increase collagen, DNA, skin thickness and elasticity.

Rhytidectomy Surgical procedure which rejuvenates the face by tightening the underlying musculature, removing excess fat deposits and redraping sagging skin of the lower face and neck. Also called a facelift.

Rosacea Acne-like skin condition characterised by a flush/blush reaction of skin, usually on the face and neck.

Salicylic acid A mild acid that encourages the sloughing of dead skin cells by stimulating the peeling of the top layer of skin and the opening of plugged follicles. Also called beta hydroxy acid.

Saline Salt water, commonly used as a filler for breast implants and in the course of administering intravenous fluids.

Scleral show Lower eyelid retraction, which exposes the sclera (white part of the eyeball) below the pupil.

Sclerotherapy The injection of one of several solutions through a small needle directly into a vein to cause it to collapse.

Sebaceous glands Oil-producing glands at the base of every sebaceous hair follicle (or pore).

Seborrheic keratoses A benign form of skin tumour that commonly appears after the age of 40.

Sebum Oil, fatty acids and wax naturally produced by sebaceous glands and expelled up through the hair shaft and on to the skin to keep it soft and pliable.

Sepsis A reaction of the body to bacteria that circulate in the blood, characterised by chills and fever.

Septum The separating wall in the nose between the left and right nasal passages.

Seroma A collection of clear fluid that may occur under the skin following surgery.

Silastic sac A sac made of rubber and silicone, often filled with silicone or salt solution.

Silicone A synthetic substance used in a gel-like form in silicone breast implants, in a liquid injectable form for facial areas and in other medical devices.

Skin cancer A malignant growth on the skin.

Sloughing Part of the skin's natural renewal process, sloughing is the act of shedding dead skin cells to make room for new ones.

SMAS The superficial musculoaponeurotic system (SMAS) is a layer of tissue that covers the deeper structures in the cheek area and touches the superficial muscle covering the lower face and neck called the platysma.

SPF (sun protection factor) A scale used to rate the level of protection sunscreens provide.

Spinal block A form of anaesthesia that numbs the lower two-thirds of the body.

Squamous cell carcinoma A type of skin cancer usually found on sun-exposed skin.

Steroid Injectable cortisone (e.g. Celestone, Kenalog), a powerful anti-inflammatory medication used to reduce swelling.

Stratum corneum The top dead layer of skin above the epidermis that acts as a physical barrier between the lower skin cells and the outside.

Striae Stretch marks caused by thinning of the underlying skin layer (dermis) that appear first as red lines, then darken and gradually flatten to form shiny white streaks.

Subglandular Under the gland, typically of the breast.

Submental Referring to the area below the chin.

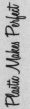

Subpectoral Also called submuscular, referring to the area below the pectoralis muscle where a breast implant may be placed.

Subperiosteal A term for a procedure in which all tissues are separated from the underlying bone structure (of, say, a brow or face), considered more invasive.

Sunblock A physical sunscreen or a barrier against the sun's ultraviolet rays.

Tazarotene A prescription topical retinoid (vitamin A derivative) for treating psoriasis, acne and photo ageing.

Tear trough The under-eye area and above the nose that often appears dark or discoloured.

Thread veins (telangiectasias) Dilated or broken blood vessels near the surface of the skin.

Tiplasty A nose augmentation or reduction procedure concerning primarily the nasal tip.

Tissue engineering The science of the production of human tissue ex vivo (outside the human body), as in growing cartilage in tissue culture.

Tissue expansion A technique in which skin or other tissue is stretched using inflatable balloons, as in breast reconstruction.

Tissue glue See Fibrin sealant.

Tragus A small extension of the auricular cartilage of the ear, anterior to the external meatus.

TRAM flap A breast reconstruction method whereby a flap of abdominal fat and skin is moved to the chest wall to form a newly reconstructed breast. TRAM is an acronym for transverse rectus abdominis myuocutaneous.

Tretinoin Synthetic vitamin A, tretinoin is the active ingredient in retinoids, which help renew skin-cell turnover and unplug pores.

Transaxillary An incision placed under the arm for access during surgery, as in breast augmentation.

Transumbilical An approach whereby the incision is placed in the umbilicus (belly button) through which breast implants may be moved into position.

Trichloroacetic acid (TCA) A colourless crystalline compound used topically as a peeling solution.

Tumescent A method of anaesthesia whereby large volumes of local anaesthetic and saline solution are injected to swell the area to be operated on.

Twilight anaesthetic Conscious sedation, also called monitored anaesthesia care.

Ultrasound Application of a sound wave, a mechanical vibration of more than 16,000 cycles per second.

Umbilicus Belly button or navel.

Undermining Surgical separation of tissues from their underlying structures.

UVA light A long wavelength (320 to 400 nanometres) of ultraviolet light that deeply penetrates the skin, affecting both the epidermis and dermis.

UVB light A wavelength (290 to 320 nanometres) of ultraviolet light that affects primarily the epidermis.

Vector The direction of pull, as in facelifting etc.

Vermillion border The external pinkish-to-red area of the upper and lower lips.

Wavelength The distance between a given point on one wave cycle and the corresponding point on the next successive wave cycle.

Xyclocaine See Lidocaine.

YAG Abbreviation for yttrium aluminium garnet, a crystal used in some types of lasers.

American Academy of Dermatology
www.aad.org
American Academy of Facial Plastic and Reconstructive Surgery
www.aafprs.org
American Society for Aesthetic Plastic Surgery
www.surgery.org
American Society for Dermatologic Surgery
www.asds.net
American Society of Plastic Surgeons
www.plasticsurgery.org
Association of Anaesthetists
www.aagbi.org
British Academy of Cosmetic Dentistry
www.bacd.com
British Association of Cosmetic Doctors
www.cosmeticdoctors.co.uk
British Association of Dermatologists (British Cosmetic Dermatology Group)
www.bad.org.uk
British Association of Oral and Maxillofacial Surgeons
www.baoms.org.uk
British Association of Otorhinolaryngologists
www.entuk.org
British Association of Plastic, Reconstructive and Aesthetic Plastic Surgeons
www.baaps.org.uk
British Association of Aesthetic Plastic Surgeons
www.bapras.co.uk

British Oculoplastic Surgery Society
www.bopss.org
European Academy of Facial Plastic Surgery
www.eafps.org
European Association of Plastic Surgeons
www.euraps.org
European Society for Laser Dermatology
www.esld.org
European Society of Plastic, Reconstructive and Aesthetic Plastic Surgery
www.espras.org
General Medical Council
www.gmc-uk.org
Healthcare Commission
www.healthcarecommission.org.uk
International Society of Plastic Surgeons
www.isaps.org
Royal College of Anaesthetists
www.rcoa.ac.uk
Wendy Lewis & Co Ltd
www.wlbeauty.com

OTHER BOOKS BY WENDY LEWIS

Nip & Talk®
e-newsletter by subscription
www.nipandtalk.com
The Lowdown on Facelifts and Other Wrinkle Remedies (Quadrille, 2000, 2001)
ISBN: 1-903845-80-7
Wrinkle Rescue (Quadrille, 2002)
ISBN: 1-903845-66-1
Figure it Out (Quadrille, 2002)
ISBN: 1-903845-68-8
Hair Affair (Quadrille, 2002)
ISBN: 1-903845-69-6
Complexion Perfection (Quadrille, 2002)
ISBN: 1-903845-67-X
Beauty Secrets (Quadrille, 2004)
ISBN: 1-84400-0931
The Beauty Battle (Laurel Glen, 2003)
ISBN: 1-59223-029-6
America's Cosmetic Doctors and Dentists (Castle Connolly Medical, 2003)
ISBN: 1-883769353, 1-883769396
America's Cosmetic Doctors and Dentists, 2nd edition (Castle Connolly Medical 2005)
ISBN: 1-883769-88-4

ACKNOWLEDGEMENTS

This is a short list of leading experts who have consistently been great sources of reliable information for me. This list is by no means complete, because of space constraints. I am very grateful to them all for their generosity in sharing their knowledge and expertise, and for their professional support. Over the past decade, there have been several individuals (you know who you are) who have attempted to silence my voice as a patient advocate. To them, I can only say that I am still here and thriving.

Dr Tina Alster, Dr Benjamin Ascher, Dr Diane Berson, Dr Thomas Biggs, Dr Fredric Brandt, Dr Allastair Carruthers, Dr Jean Carruthers, Dr Bernard Cornette de St Cyr, Mr Dai Davies, Dr Javier De Benito, Dr Steven Fagien, Dr Timothy Flynn, Dr Peter Bela Fodor, Dr Bryan Forley, Dr Nelly Gauthier, Dr Melanie Grossman, Mr Rajiv Grover, Dr Joseph Gryskiewicz, Dr Per Heden, Dr Judith Hellman, Dr David Hidalgo, Dr Dennis Hurwitz, Mr Chris Inglefield, Mr Barry M. Jones, Dr Michael Kaminer, Dr Arielle Kauvar, Dr Laurence Kirwan, Dr Jana Klauer, Dr Albert Lefkouits, Ms Elaine Linker, Dr Gregg Lituchy, Dr Z. Paul Lorenc, Dr Nicholas Lowe, Dr Marc Lowenberg, Dr Stephen Mandy, Dr Timothy J. Marten, Dr Alan Matarasso, Dr Seth Matarasso, Mr Basim Matti, Dr G. Patrick Maxwell, Dr Bryan Mendelson, Dr Nicolas Metaxotos, Dr Gary Monheit, Dr Foad Nahai, Dr Rhoda Narins, Dr Amy Newberger, Dr Malcolm Paul, Dr Steven Pearlman, Mr Nicholas Percival, Dr Gerald Pitman, Dr Rita Rakus, Dr Samieh Rizk, Dr Rod Rohrich, Dr Thomas Romo III, Dr Mark G. Rubin, Dr Gregory Ruff, Dr Joca Sampaio-Goes, Dr Scott Spear, Dr James Stuzin, Dr Dean Toriumi, Dr Donald Wood-Smith

INDEX

Bold refers to main entries in text.

Plastic Makes Perfect

Wendy Lewis is an international image enhancement coach and beauty guru, renowned as 'one of the world's leading authorities on cosmetic surgery'. Dubbed The Knife Coach®, she writes a popular column for *YOU* magazine in the *Mail on Sunday*, where she answers readers' queries about all cosmetic beauty topics, and she is a frequent contributor to *Financial Times'* How to Spend It and Russian *Vogue*. She appears regularly on television, including BBC, GMTV and CNN, is a sought-after radio guest, and is frequently featured in numerous magazines and newspapers including *Vogue, Elle, InStyle, Marie Claire, Time, The New York Times, Sunday Times* (London) and the London *Evening Standard*.

Wendy Lewis & Co Ltd is based in New York City and Ms Lewis travels to London and Paris to see private clients; she also conducts telephone consultations from all over the world. Her personal e-newsletter, Nip & Talk®, covers global trends and newsy tips, and is offered by subscription on her website. Ask The Beauty Junkie® is the website's signature feature, which attracts visitors from all over the world who pose questions. In 2007, The Knife Coach® celebrates her ten-year anniversary, and *Plastic Makes Perfect* marks her tenth book.

New York office telephone: 001-212-861-6148
Email: wlbeauty@aol.com
Website: www.wlbeauty.com

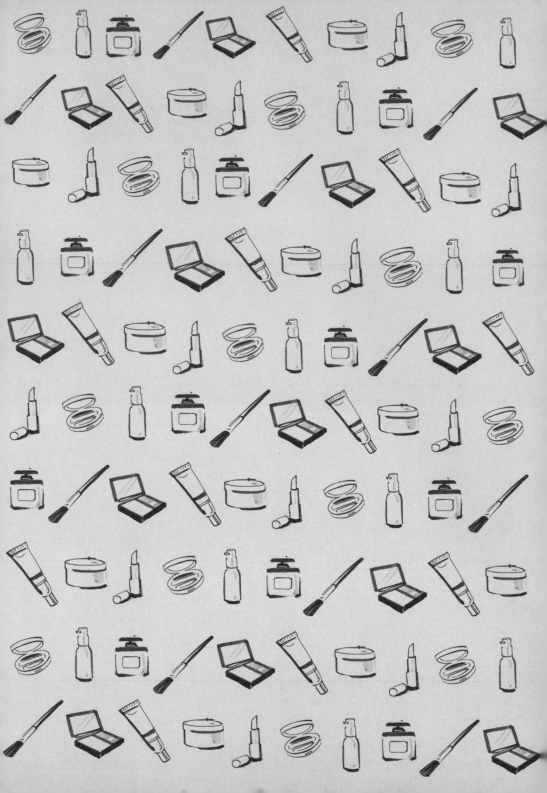